"A must-read for everyone touched
by disease or trauma."
— Bob Proctor

"Life is unpredictable. Dr. Barr's book offers a unique
framework to guide you through those times."
— Ari Brown, M.D., pediatrician
and author of the Baby 411 book series

"Lori Barr is that rare M.D. who is willing to consider
answers not yet fully accepted by the establishment. Read
her book, and you'll be encouraged that rigorous science
and education don't always destroy imagination and the
human spirit. Dr. Barr is a brilliant scientist who cares
about people far more than she cares about protocol."
— Roy H. Williams, New York Times bestselling
author of The Wizard of Ads trilogy

"Dr. Barr's book prepares you to handle the unexpected
by using one of the most powerful tools possible — your
own mind. Powerful, insightful, and necessary!"
— Lorie Marrero, creator of ClutterDiet.com and
author of The Clutter Diet: The Skinny on Organizing
Your Home and Taking Control of Your Life

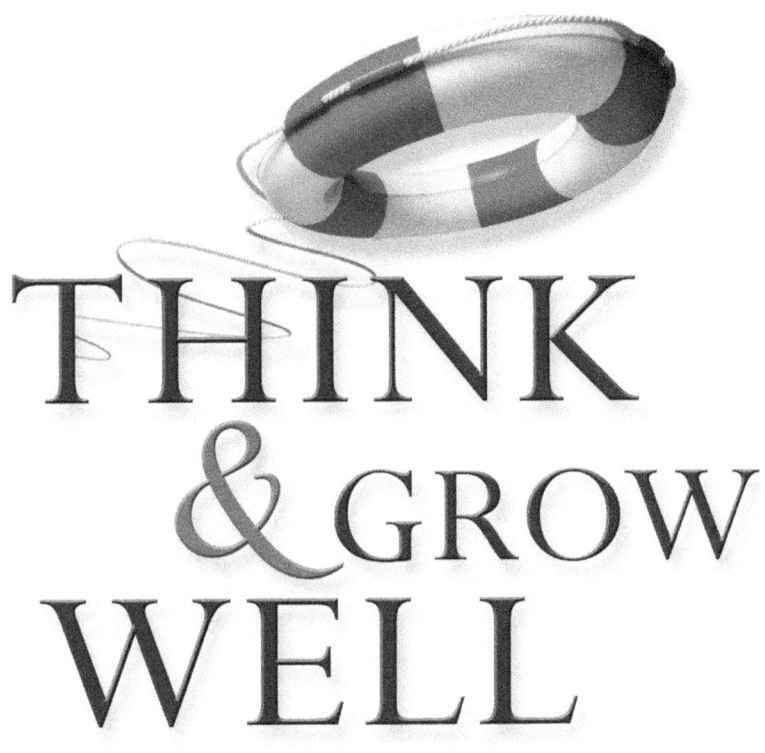

THINK & GROW WELL

CREATE AND PRESERVE YOUR TOTAL HEALTH

LORI L. BARR, M. D.

© 2014 by Lori L. Barr, M.D.
All Rights Reserved. This book may not be reproduced in whole or in part, by any means, in any physical or digital format, without written consent of the publisher.

www.thinkandgrowwell.com

This book is written as a source of information only. The information included in the book should by no means be considered a substitute for the advice, decisions, or judgement of the reader's physician or other professional advisor.

All efforts have been made to ensure the accuracy of the information contained in this book as of the date published. The author and the publisher expressly disclaim responsibility for any adverse affects arising from the use or application of information contained herein.

Cover, layout and graphics by Bella Guzmán, Highwire Creative
Portrait photo: Steve Armstrong
Illustrations by Robin Kressbach, The Robin's Nest

ISBN-13: 978-1494961541
ISBN-10: 1494961547

Other Published Works by the Author

Books
Handbook of Pediatric Imaging
Journal to Think and Grow Well

Audio
Mental Tattoos
Four Pillars of Parenting
Think and Grow Well

Chapters
"Neurosonography," in *Ultrasound Clinics of North America, 2009*

"Mental Tattoos," in *DNA of Success Stories*

"Pediatric Bone Diseases," in *Essentials of Musculoskeletal Imaging*

"Intraoperative Ultrasound of the Brain," in *Intraoperative, Laparoscopic and Endoluminal Ultrasound*

"Neonatal Cranial Ultrasound," in *Radiology Clinics of North America, 1999*

"Mentors;" "Using a Computer to Improve Your Efficiency;" and "Nurturing Personal Relationships;" in *Survival Guide for Women Radiologists: The AAWR Pocket Mentor*

"Ultrasonography of the Pediatric and Adolescent Pelvis," in *Gynecological Imaging*

"Pediatrics," in *The Yearbook of Ultrasound, 1996*

"Elbow," in *Clinics in Diagnostic Ultrasound: Musculoskeletal Ultrasound*

Dedication

To Gene Dent and Greg Sterling, men remembered for service to others and untimely passage to the place beyond.

Contents

Preface xi
Foreword xvii
Introduction 1
1 Mind Tamed, Life Saved (Avoid Sudden Death) 7
2 The Illness Wears Prada (Strip Away Malaise) 17
3 Why Did I Do That? (Cure the Unexplainable) 31
4 Where Did I Go? (Find Your Purpose) 45
5 Reset Your Ease-o-Stat™ (Nullify Stress) 59
6 The Dance with Disease (Face Illness Without Fear) 67
7 From Mission Impossible to Mission Accomplished
   (Kindle Passion) 81
8 Time for the Life Preserver (Save Yourself First) 93
9 Spiritual Mastery (Live Up to Your Word) 103
10 Physical Mastery (Fat Off Fast) 113
11 The Scientific Establishment Versus You
   (Examine Your Doctor) 123
12 The Gift of Appreciation (Bottomless Gratitude) 135
13 Let Go (Kick Habits) 145
14 Cross the Finish Line (Go Out in Style) 157
Epilogue 167
Appendix 1 Make an Ease-o-Stat™ 171
Afterword 175
Acknowledgements 177
Bibliography 179
Index 187

Preface

This book provides a skill path for new habits that can create unconditional vitality and preserve total health. This means you will learn simple solutions to common problems, transitions people face as they strive to live as well as possible. It differs from other books by equally qualified experts in two important ways. First off, it puts the control of your wellness back into the hands that matter most: your hands. Second, the combination of stories, actions, and exploration help you develop new thoughts, feelings, and actions that get results fast.

You need this book if you feel that your body has let you down, or if you feel as if you have no more energy left for yourself. It is written for individuals who want to understand why the body responds one way when they think it should do something else. It is written for those who admire friends and family living vibrantly and who want to move toward radical vibrancy in their own lives. It is written for people who know they are more than just a body.

It is written for people like Mr. Fernandez, a healthy Hispanic man. Sweating and squirming on the exam table he awaits the news from his physician, who is frowning, his brow furrowed. "Mr. Fernandez" the doctor says, "your biopsy results are back, and I am sorry to be the bearer of bad news. You have prostate cancer."

No matter what words follow, Mr. Fernandez will not hear them. Mr. Fernandez's mind has just received a shocking jolt, and it is in a state of chaos. Very few diseases have the power to immobilize the mind as cancer does. Although "cancer" is just a word, when given life in a mind full of fear and doubt, it grows in strength. Is it any wonder that this disease is empowered to usurp resources from healthy tissues and spread unchecked throughout the body? In the weeks that follow, Mr. Fernandez and millions of others like him continue in a state of confusion. They constantly worry about three recurring themes and ask themselves three questions:

- Is my tumor removable?
- Has my tumor spread?
- Does this cancer signal my demise?

When diagnosed with cancer the next step for most individuals is imaging to determine the extent of disease. They may undergo a computer-assisted tomography (CAT) scan. Then a radiologist, like me interprets the images. We radiologists are physicians who train for years to understand the intricate anatomy and function of the body and to master the safest, most effective means of imaging the body to either diagnose or treat diseases. The radiologist speaks with the doctor and describes the size, shape, and location of the tumor; surrounding structures compromised by the tumor; and signs of distant disease or metastasis.

Curiosity peaks at the thought of forbidden images of oneself. All humans are fascinated with pictures of themselves but especially with pictures they rarely have a chance to glimpse. The subconscious mind is at peak attention because of this fascination and curiosity. Many newly diagnosed individuals who undergo medical imaging are curious about their insides and want to see the pictures. Then it happens: the subconscious mind immediately assimilates the CAT scan picture containing both tumor and patient—along with the worry, fear, and doubt associated with the cancer diagnosis—and makes a memory. This is mentally stored in the "Very Important Files" because there is so much curiosity, emotion, and time spent thinking about this dire disease.

Once a memory like this is filed, it is very difficult to see yourself apart from your diagnosis. Consider it a mental tattoo. A tattoo is a shock to your body as it happens, and it hurts for quite some time. Ink is injected into the skin layers, and when those layers spread, the sensitive nerve endings are negatively stimulated. It hurts! Skin sloughs off over time, and when scarring subsides, the art remains. It seems almost permanent. With proper attention to detail, both tattoos and memories of a shocking diagnosis entwined with our very being can be removed.

Perhaps you have heard people say things like this:

- "I am a diabetic."
- "I am an epileptic."
- "I am anorexic."

These individuals are not who they say they are. To the subconscious mind, each statement reinforces a picture of disease, a mental tattoo rather than health. *Think and Grow Well* is written for both patients and health-care colleagues. The book provides a framework so that you are able to recognize and act decisively in the moments that define your health. With it, readers teach themselves to become mentally and physically prepared before trauma strikes so that they can live lives filled with uncommon depth and passion.

Think and Grow Well teaches you to exercise your will, just as you would your biceps, so that you stay well. In the chapters that follow, explore how the mind works; examine how you achieve your results; and develop strategies to help see yourself as the person you are instead of any disease you may have.

I first began working in hospitals in New Orleans when I was 12. Before becoming a doctor, I was a volunteer, then an emergency room receptionist, then a medical student, then an intern, a resident in diagnostic radiology, and a fellow in pediatric radiology. I then spent ten years working up the academic ranks in Cincinnati, Ohio. Many people passed through these institutions, most with mental tattoos and a few people who, in spite of their diseases or injuries, never seemed to succumb to low-end thoughts. These rare patients got out of the hospital more quickly and required less medication. They were fun to work with as their vitality grew. Individuals like these recognize health opportunities where their choices make a difference. They train themselves to take advantage of opportunities. They are fascinating, and I imagined I was on them, but it turns out I was wrong. (More on that later in this book.)

As a radiologist, however, reading thousands of imaging studies each year, I'd learned to recognize patterns. I applied that skill to the study of these individuals, the ones who either never seemed to get a mental tattoo or the ones who had learned to remove them. These individuals tapped in to a fourth aspect of their being that went beyond body, mind and spirit-awareness. After recognizing this trait, I wrote this book to teach others how to develop the framework necessary to become resilient. The mind likes to latch on to pictures, so visualize the framework as the beginning of a rope. The rope represents your life. These individuals anchor themselves by strengthening the four strands of their being: spiritual, mental, physical, and conscious awareness. They strengthen each individual strand, determine a weaving pattern, and take meaningful action to begin the braiding process of their lifeline. They braid their lifeline strengthening the rope.

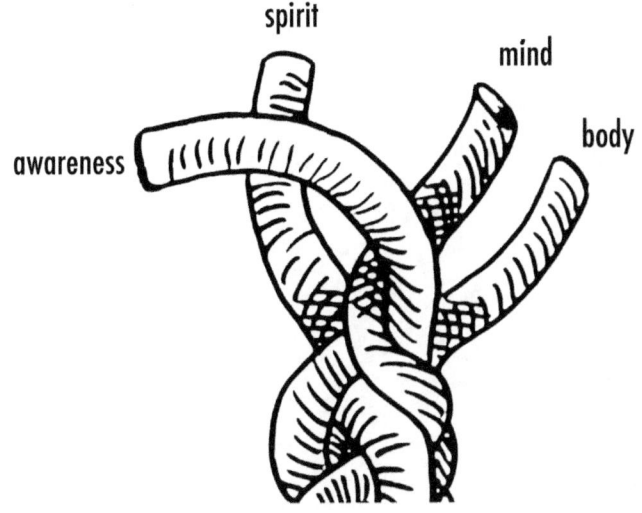

The chapters of *Think and Grow Well* each correspond to one of the four strands of being, and this is graphically identified at the beginning of each chapter. The chapters are arranged to braid a pattern for the start or reinforcement of your lifeline. Learn the steps for creating an orderly pattern of vitality using all four strands. As you begin to enjoy the more vibrant you, recognize how much more complete you are with all aspects of your being in action than if you chose to leave a few unrecognized. My goal in writing is to give you the tools you need to become the most vibrant being you possibly can be so you recognize your unique purpose and have the best chance in the world to create the relationships you need to fulfill it. I have successfully applied this in my own life, as have countless patients in my care. If you are ready to move to a place in life where you are in top condition and you have the awareness to know what instances really make a difference in health, read and be well.

Foreword

I was delighted and somewhat surprised when Lori Barr asked me to write a foreword for her new book on harnessing the mind and the spirit to achieve physical health and emotional balance. When I learned that Lori started a nonmedical consulting business outside of her radiology practice and had a book on helping people think through and prepare for medical crises before they occur, I was curious to know why she added this ambitious mission to her already very full and busy life. As a woman with a family, a busy medical practice imaging children in Austin, and an active spiritual life, she has more than ample opportunity to give back to others. Reflection on our time together as fellow radiology residents reminded me that Lori has always wanted to help people in this way.

Lori Barr, M.D., started her medical career at Louisiana State University School of Medicine at the age of 19. She was drawn to the field of medicine that is most devoted to diagnosis of disease, diagnostic radiology. I was fortunate to join her as first-year residents at the University of Texas Medical Branch in Galveston, Texas. We found that our paths would be intertwined for the next 25 years.

The days of a radiology resident are filled with hours of reading, talking with patients, performing complex procedures, dictating numerous reports of imaging studies, preparing lectures and case presentations, and receiving critiques from teachers and colleagues. I often left work exhausted, but Lori was able to accomplish all of the required tasks and leave the hospital with plenty of energy, eager to explore different but equally interesting worlds outside of medicine. She was never content with the status quo, always seeking ways to improve her surroundings both at work and at home. Loving music, she designed a research study to evaluate whether music could be used to calm children while undergoing an ultrasound exam. She sought novel ways of sharing information, including writing a series of comic books. After residency, Lori became a faculty member at the University of Cincinnati College of Medicine, where she practiced pediatric radiology, conducted medical research, and taught for ten years. There she established herself as a talented investigator and author as well as an accomplished physician, publishing 35 scientific papers, 11 book chapters, and a textbook on pediatric imaging. While Lori's career in radiology involves helping to diagnose existing disease, this text reveals her strong desire to help prevent pain and disease. Like many professional women, she has struggled to balance her goals, desires, and responsibilities. Through it all, she always has time to share with her family, her friends, and her cats. This book is her way of sharing herself with you.

The format of *Think and Grow Well* is a reflection of Lori's approach to life. This is not a book that strives to present a list of rules or guidelines that should be applied to everyone's lives uniformly, but rather it describes exercises that one can use to strengthen one's entire infrastructure. We used programmed texts in medical school to learn to perform tasks such as interpreting chest x-rays or electrocardiograms. Lori takes the same learning tool and applies it to the more abstract concepts of grappling with disease. Lori uses many practical examples from her own life experience to demonstrate the effects of thoughts and emotions on the physical self, and she is clear that each person must create his or her own unique path. Lori's exercises build on ideas proposed by other authors and on scientific research, and she provides useful references for further study. I especially appreciate the discussion of the importance of gratitude, a concept that cannot be overemphasized. The text provides ample pages for notes, supporting the concept that writing your thoughts brings enlightenment. Like all good mentors, she shares experiences and ideas, encourages action, and applies gentle pressure on the reader to complete the expected tasks. Lori stresses that we are responsible for our own health and challenges us all to get up and take charge of our lives. For those willing to participate, this book can open the door to a life of self-discovery and wellness.

Susan D. John, M.D.
Professor and Chair of Diagnostic Radiology
University of Texas Medical School at Houston
Houston, Texas

Introduction

Just around the time of my birth, my father was in the United States Coast Guard, assigned to a cutter anchored in Chesapeake Bay and riding out a hurricane. In the middle of the night, he heard a heart-stopping alarm. The captain announced, "All hands prepare to abandon ship!" Each officer and sailor had been assigned a particular task to secure the ship. Then the seamen were to report to the deck near the lifeboats and don their life preservers.

My father served as an engineer. When he heard the order, he secured a door to make a compartment deep in the ship's bowels watertight so that she might stay afloat even if abandoned. When he reported to deck, he was slapped by the wind's wet hands and sloshed about getting into his life preserver. As he told me this story, he stopped to add, "I then saw the scariest thing I'd ever seen." Looking into the past, he continued, "A much larger ship had broken from its mooring and was drifting into us sideways. She was headed right for us, and there was nothing we could do." Daddy returned to the present. "I don't know how many times during my career I performed that abandon-ship drill, but this was the real thing."

The more he told me about this frightening experience, the more I realized that sea analogies are particularly relevant to the principles of steering your own health. When a man falls overboard, he is thrown a lifeline. When you learn to take control of the way you view wellness obstacles, you throw yourself a lifeline. Through self-discipline, you weave the strands of your being: your mind, your spiritual nature, conscious awareness, and your physical body into a strong rope of hope so you don't drown in disease. You think and grow well.

I wonder if that is what my father's crew did. He stood on the deck with the rest of the crew ready to abandon ship. The tanker careened sideways toward their vessel, and because they already had done everything they had prepared themselves to do in that critical instant, the only thing left to do was to trust, keep watch, and pray. Just before the tanker broke them to pieces, the tanker's crew managed to get their vessel underway and used their current momentum to back away from the collision course. The front of the tanker narrowly missed the cutter as they tiptoed across the angry deep. Everyone cheered. They thought and acted their way out of an impossible situation because they practiced drills that allowed them to take decisive action in the critical moment.

You've heard of fire drills and of disaster drills; why not consider this a will drill? Practice at skills that help you to develop the will, one of your most important intellectual faculties.

How is this accomplished for you in the chapters ahead?

There are 14 chapters in *Think and Grow Well*. Focus on the exercises in one chapter for a minimum of 21 days.

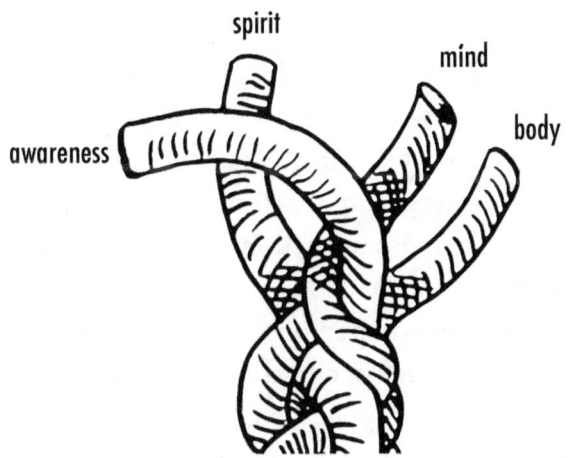

At the beginning of each chapter, a diagram highlights the part of yourself the chapter activities will strengthen: body, mind, spirit, or awareness. A "Lesson Summary" follows. Next, read a story that teaches the main chapter lesson. If you desire to find your own story, the companion activity guide, *Journal to Think and Grow Well*, is cross-referenced.

I've included three nautical symbols throughout this guide as points of reference for you, alerting you to an action interlude, action step, or a deeper understanding, all listed as follows.

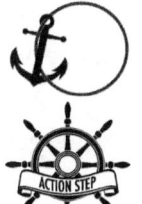

Action Interlude
Stop and perform the task.

Action Step
Stop and perform the task at the close of each chapter.

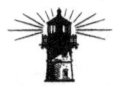

Deeper Understanding
Digital and physical recommendations for continued exploration.

If your goal is to be able to make a difference in your own vitality by acting decisively in the moments where your actions matter with regard to health, then you must do more than read a book. This is your personal journey of your thoughts, feelings, and actions that occur as you study. Thoughts, feelings, and actions form one's attitude, so this is no idle exercise.

The tasks in the companion activity guide, *Journal to Think and Grow Well,* are specifically designed to assist you in accessing the vast untapped potential of your marvelous mind. Performing the tasks builds persistence. Success in these small actions will help you to build a storehouse of faith in these ideas. That faith and your experiences will be available to you whenever you meet a new challenge and need a quick infusion of energy. That is the whole idea behind thinking to grow well.

Action interludes and steps strengthen your inquisitive nature. This is critical for rapid transition from old paradigms to new paradigms. A paradigm is a set of habits that is so engrained that you act without thinking. Sometimes old paradigms, groups of old habits, no longer serve you. The action steps are designed to provide spaced repetition of new ideas so that you quickly form new habits that serve you better.

Finally, a list of recommendations for gaining deeper understanding closes each chapter. Expand your understanding of certain concepts that were introduced in the chapter and are beyond the scope of *Journal to Think and Grow Well.* In general, books or digital media are referenced. This does not mean you have to read that exact book. For instance, I frequently reference the Bible and, because I am a Christian, point especially to the New Testament for inspiration.

Yet I recognize that other religious texts may hold special meaning for you. and I encourage you to pursue them with conviction. Still, because I have found particular value in the resources I recommend, I hope you'll explore them. Search for the authors online, explore their websites, or watch movie trailers or online video clips. Let your intuition and spiritual practice guide you on the use of these resources. Investigate them, and get in step with a new way of thinking. Let yourself meet the people, places, and things introduced, and list those items worthy of your attention.

Whether you are reading *Think and Grow Well* for yourself or for someone you dearly love, get comfortable, take a deep breath, and set your intention on learning this framework and mastering the skills you need to see your true self, your perfect self, your multidimensional self. This is a programmed text. Just like any disaster drill, there is an orderly way to proceed through this will-drill. Follow the plan and practice the material. In exchange, I affirm that my heart's desire is to help you become whole so that you may live your life's purpose as intended. One idea is all it takes to change your world.

Chapter 1
Mind Tamed, Life Saved
(Avoid Sudden Death)

A human being is part of a whole, called by us the universe, a part limited in time and space. He experiences himself, his thoughts and feelings, as something separated from the rest, a kind of optical delusion of his consciousness. This delusion is a kind of prison for us, restricting us to our personal desires and to affection for a few persons nearest us. Our task must be to free ourselves from this prison by widening our circles of compassion to embrace all living creatures and the whole of nature in its beauty.
—Albert Einstein

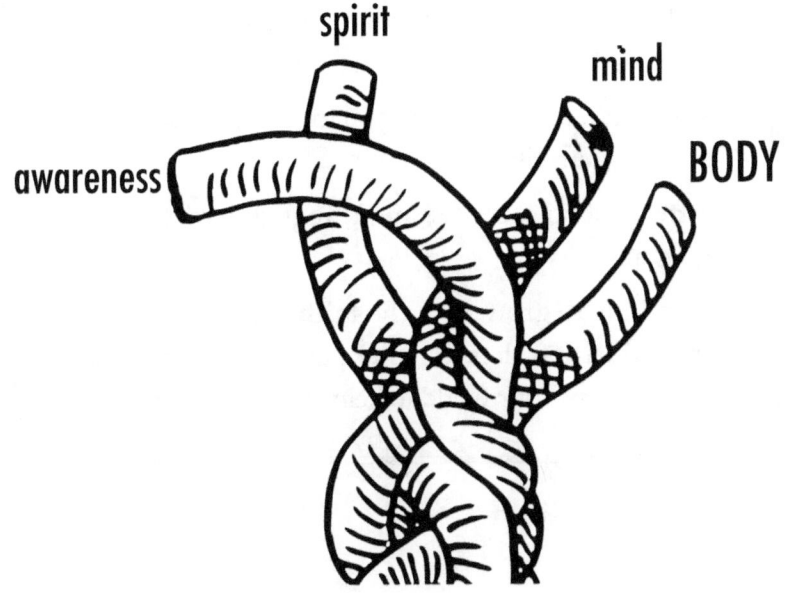

Lesson Summary

Malady alert: if you haven't had a personal "wake up, this is your life" call yet, use this as an opportunity to go through a dry run and really prepare yourself for when the time comes. You taste what lies ahead in this will- drill; now begin to master the basic survival skills you need to deal with diseases.

Here are the steps you must take to move through the fear:

- **Presence of mind** gives you the personal power to make a difference in the outcome.

- Decide on a **definite goal**.

- Act immediately and boldly with a **grateful heart**. This leads to unexpected success.

- Apply the skills that allow you to tap into **reserves** beyond yourself.

- **Attract** people, places, and things that make the goal a reality.

- Continue to grow with the **faith** that as a unique individual you alone can make the difference needed right now in your world to help so many others.

Nate's Story

Breathless and sweating the offensive tackle for the Northlake High School Riders listens to the rundown of the 75-yard push the offense made to tie the game against Cumberland at 7–7. As Nate sits on the bench and talks with a good friend, the cold, wet towel on his neck fails to relieve the burning inside. The 88 degrees feels like a wet sauna after the big push. Nate fades and falls backward off the bench; feet lag behind; eyes roll up. He is unconscious. Nate's heart stops. One minute, Nate lives the dream of a winning senior year team, with plans for college and the NFL; the next minute, his life slips away on the grass field sidelines.

Two doctors, an orthopedist and a nephrologist, watch Nate from the stands. They respond immediately with professionalism, competence, and courageous decisions that help Nate rejoin the living. Timely use of an automated external defibrillator (AED) changes his ineffective heart rhythm back to one that sustains his life. The two doctors respond with love and compassion, for they are also Nate's parents. Nate lives today because of the ability of his parents to tame their emotions and fully use their professional training for the benefit of their own son. Nate gives hope to many others by his political activism on a state level as he tells his story to increase awareness about the value of AEDs in schools.

Presence of Mind Gives You Personal Power

Nate's story is a good example of the untimely nature of many illnesses and of the benefits of mind training so that you are prepared whenever trauma arises. Disease tends to strike when you least expect it, either when you are at your peak or perhaps when you think you are beaten down to the bottom. No one—regardless of race, sex, creed, or ethnicity—is immune. You can be a healthy football star like Nate and still quickly face your mortality. Just as we all benefit by emergency preparedness training, such as chest compressions and AED use, we benefit from learning the steps it takes to tame our emotions or reactivity and free our minds for ordered, productive action. This is the first lesson of *Think and Grow Well*. Is it easy to tame your mind? The process is simple and easy to understand, and few individuals take the time to commit the desire, faith, and perseverance necessary to make substantial changes in the way they think. Most people are quite content to go through the motions of life. They exist on a lower level of awareness, either fully consumed with the process of survival or fully content to follow the herd. But it is worth your effort to master the workings of your mind and the effects on your physique and your reality.

Why go to the trouble to train and tame your mind? The reasons fall into three categories: spiritual, intellectual, and physical. The foremost spiritual reason is that sometime before we die, we tend to recognize our unique nature throughout the entire time-space continuum that we call the universe. No one else is just like you. Nothing could be worse than the realization of a life frittered away on inconsequential activities without regard for why you were put here on earth.

As humans, a personal nonphysical component, our soul, ties us to the universal spiritual nature of all creation and its origin. *Spirit* is always for fullness and expansion, for creation. We are here as creators. What do we create? Each of us creates our reality, and in the process shapes our personal existence and the worlds of today and tomorrow.

How does that occur? Through the medium of the

intellect, we receive or formulate ideas; refer them to the powerhouse of our mind, the subconscious; and give them energy and substrate so that they begin to take form and create a vibration that resonates within and without our bodies. Other people, places, and situations in harmony with this vibration are attracted. When the mind is tamed, this process occurs naturally and unfettered. This is when we truly recognize ourselves at our best.

Unfortunately, most people fail to understand this key process. They unwittingly use the power of their mind to their detriment, and that reflects a third, very *physical* reason to tame the mind. The actions taken spiritually and intellectually directly cause physical effects. A growing body of scientific evidence indicates that the way we perceive our social status, health, wealth, and well-being correlates with diseases such as hypertension, viral infections, colds, chronic lung disease, and weakening of the immune defenses.

Self Image and the Physical Condition

The way we perceive ourselves, our self-image also impacts the environment we create around us. For example, we know without a doubt that pesticides contribute to increased congenital anomalies, allergies, and chronic diseases, yet why do we think we cannot afford organic foods? We know that fiber supplementation can decrease cholesterol, improve bowel function, and decrease the likelihood of colon cancer, yet why do we refuse to use a fiber supplement or change our diet? Instead, we rely on prescription medication to take away the symptoms and mask the underlying disease.

Why is that? In one phrase, the answer to these questions is self-image, our perception of our self. The way we think about ourselves influences the actions we take with our bodies. Consider the fiber. First, our self-image causes us to think things like, "If the doctor didn't prescribe it, who am I to think that I know better than he does?" Next, we think, "If the insurance won't pay for it, it is a luxury I do not deserve or cannot afford." Our self-image, the way we perceive ourselves, is the major reason we fail to act on many opportunities that we attract.

Act Immediately

Look again at the title of this chapter. Tame is verb, and *Think and Grow Well* is a call to action. Throughout each chapter, action interludes invite you to stop, reflect, choose, and act. If you choose to "read" *Think and Grow Well*, you will increase your knowledge. Beware! Knowledge is not enough to make substantial changes in your life. You must act and infuse your subconscious mind with the new teaching. This occurs through spaced repetition. If, instead, you choose to "do" *Think and Grow Well* (read, reflect, act, reflect), you substantially increase your level of awareness with regard to your vitality and existence. Mind taming, as Nate's parents demonstrate, is a process of self-discipline that every human being alive has equal opportunity to master. Most of the time we come to mastery only through the use of a guide, a mentor, or a coach. A coach is a person who has considerable experience in reflecting our reality back to us and helping us shape our future. We must choose the role of willing student: ready to listen, eager to apply the principles, happy to learn and to grow. Consider me your coach for now, and make the commitment to become a serious student of your mind.

Action Interlude

Take five minutes right now and begin a journal of your thoughts as you start Think and Grow Well. Put yourself in the place of Nate, a young man with a new lease on life after a near-death experience, who gave up his football dreams. Or put yourself in the place of one of Nate's parents, adults with specialized knowledge faced with a personal challenge that means life or death to their child. Using your creative imagination, see, taste, smell, feel, and hear yourself in one of these roles with your current skill set. Visualize the entire scenario.

Then ask yourself some tough questions, questions like, "If I came that close to death, what would I do with the remainder of my time here?" Or, "If that was my child, how would I react?"

Look back once more at Einstein's observation, quoted at the beginning of this chapter. Ask yourself, "What kind of a prison have I placed myself in?" This is not small talk. Ask at least five hard questions, and spend at least a minute per question writing down an answer in your own handwriting or recording your answer in your own voice with an MP3 recorder or tape recorder. If you choose to type your answers on the computer, be aware that later in the book I recommend actions to be recorded in your own handwriting rather than on the computer because your subconscious mind is madly in love with you. Just like any jealous lover, your subconscious mind wants spoken words and handwritten letters from you. Your own voice and your own writing are the most influential tools you have for riding the wave of vitality.

Grow with Faith that You Make a Difference

Growing is never comfortable. Think of how your body feels when you implement a new exercise regimen. If you begin to run two miles after a period of sedentary life at the computer, two days later you notice an exquisite tenderness in muscles you didn't even know you had. The same occurs when you grow in self-awareness and when you grow into better use of your intellectual faculties, your mental muscles. The mental muscles that a will-drill flexes are imagination, intuition, memory, perception, reason, and will. You will feel uncomfortable until a new habit is established. Embrace this discomfort as a sign of growth, and move forward, even if it scares you to death.

Scared to death. That is how Nate, his parents, his teammates, his coaches, and most of the surrounding fans felt when his wake-up call came in September 2006. Presence of mind was the prevailing factor that saved his life. His parents were watching him out of love and joy. They did not sit immobilized by fear when the wake-up call came. They decided to fight, and they acted immediately. They mastered life-saving skills at an earlier time; tapped into those skills; and, through automatic recall, used those skills to carry their son through his crisis. They moved through their worst nightmare, faced their fear, and saved his life. That's what you are doing now. You are mastering life-saving skills of a different sort that you, too, will be able to rely upon when your wake-up call comes, whenever you face a trauma. We can't all be lion tamers, but we can master our minds and save lives.

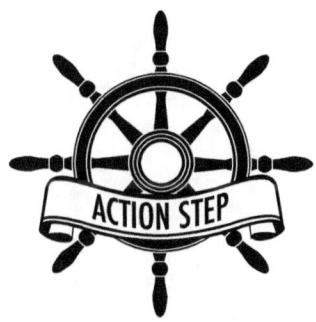

ACTION STEP

Read the book *The Death of Ivan Ilyich*, or watch the movie *Ikiru*. Take your answers to the questions from the Action Interlude above and begin to look at the people you surround yourself with in a different light. Determine which people are living with purpose and which are going through the motions. Are you living with as much purpose as you are capable?

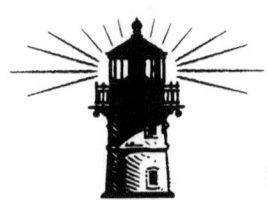

Deeper Understanding

The Death of Ivan Ilyich, Leo Tolstoy, The Editorium, West Valley City, UT, 2006.

Ikiru, 1952, movie produced by Akira Kurosawa.

"Health psychology: developing biologically plausible models linking the social world and physical health," by Miller et al., SW. *Annu Rev Psychol.* 2009; 60:501-24.

The Mind Map Book, Tony and Barry Buzan, Penguin Books, New York, NY, 1996.

"Once by the Pacific," a poem by Robert Frost, in *West Running Brook,* Henry Holt, New York, NY, 1928.

Chapter 2
The Illness Wears Prada
(Strip Away Malaise)

*You better stay away from him; he'll rip your lungs out, Jim.
Huh. I'd like to meet his tailor.*
—Warren Zevon

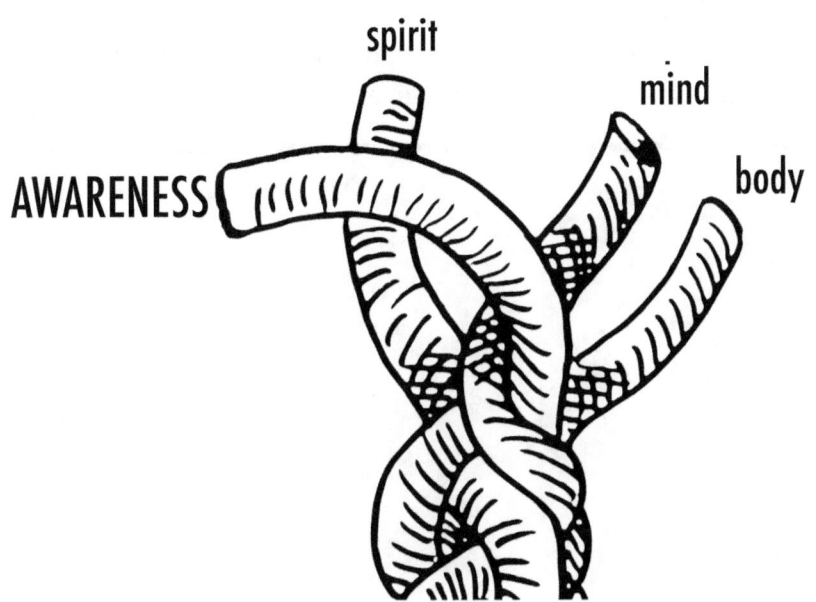

Lesson Summary

- Three uncharacteristic emotions accompany disease: worry, fear, and doubt.

- Recognition of the nonphysical portions of your being helps you to understand from whence these emotions arise.

- These emotions arise from three primary sources: your genetic programming, your environment, and your paradigms.

- Awareness to sensory triggers increases when one reflects on past shocking events.

Darcie's Story

"This turkey is just moist enough to make a great sandwich," thinks Darcie as she chews. She enjoys the new smell of the remodeled kitchen that mingles with the turkey. Suddenly, tingly prickles assault a spot of mayonnaise and black pepper at the right corner of her mouth. Her eyes widen. She sighs in disbelief that it has started again: her tongue feels like a slug sliding over a grain of salt. A dentist's numbing needle could not have been more effective in spoiling this solitary meal.

This is not supposed to be happening. The doctor said the swelling and numbness were side effects of medicine she used to take, so six months ago she had stopped all of her medicines, and it had not happened in all that time. She quickly rises and moves to a place of safety. She knows that she has only a few minutes before the darkness comes and the world slips away. Darcie is afraid. The last time she was in her car, luckily in her driveway, when her neighbor found her. Her tongue feels like a balloon nursing a helium tank. She calls her husband.

"It ith happening again!" she musters, and speaks as clearly as she can as her tongue swells. "I hope it isn't a stroke," she thinks, because strokes run in her family.

"Don't worry," he reassures, "this is no different from the last spell."

Tears stream from her eyes as a blinding pain seems to pierce her skull base. Even though she has not fallen, her head hurts as if the floor reached up and smacked her. From the safety of her pillow, she quietly squeezes back the tears of frustration as she wonders if she will ever be truly free of this mysterious pain. Who is this unknown assailant robbing her of her vitality?

Worry, Fear and Doubt

An illness, conjuring emotions as powerful as an otherworldly specter, has just paid Darcie a visit. He is a tall, brooding stranger in dark yet stylish trappings. He and all of his relatives, all manner of diseases, injuries, and illness clothe themselves in the same stylish garb. Illness stalks the unaware in a kilt of fear, a cloak of worry and a hood of doubt that aids the illness as it abducts vitality. Just as Darcie struggles with her feelings (she still doesn't have an answer), so does every other individual who experiences unnamed diseases.

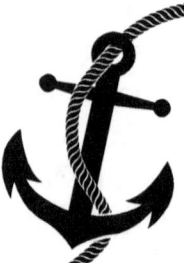

Action Interlude

Reread Darcie's story and identify the following:

What did she fear?

What caused her worry?

What did she doubt about herself?

Why are diseases so frightening?

You Are More Than Just a Body

The main reason we become victims in this cycle is that as modern, self-absorbed, fashion-conscious individuals, we identify more with our bodies than we should. You are not a body; you *have* a body. It is an instrument of your being. It is yours to use for a time, just like your blunt-tipped scissors from the first grade. Your body is a tool designed to serve you for a finite time as you interact with other living beings and your world. So if you are a not a body, what exactly are you?

Your Non-Physical Self

You are a spiritual being that has unbounded potential for connection, creation, and translation. Don't believe it? Consider the effect of death. Death is the cessation of animation of the body. Within three years of our marriage, Steve and I adopted a beautiful cat that was a medical-research refugee. He had long, soft white fur with scattered beige spots and a bushy tail. His research name was Beige Tail, we called him B. T. He was the most intelligent cat of all of the cats with which I've shared time. He enhanced our lives for about ten years. During summer vacation, we left B. T. and our other cats with a pet sitter, she found B. T. unconscious in our backyard and rushed him to our veterinarian, but it was too late. He died and we never knew exactly why.

After death, B.T.'s body didn't do him any good, because all of the animation that made him so enchanting had ceased—the body is a useful tool only when animated by a well-balanced animator. What do you call the myriad of movement that animates the body? Spirit. Spirit exists completely separate from the physical realm and is always moving toward creation and expansion.

Let's continue the distinction of our nonphysical portions into a separation of soul from spirit, mind, and awareness. The soul is our individuality on the nonphysical plane of existence, whereas the spirit simply represents all of the nonphysical factors about us as animate beings. If the word *soul* causes you discomfort, *persona* or *psyche* might be other words to describe the part of our spirit that is unique to each of us as individuals. Mind is the movement that translates our energy on the spiritual level to the concrete

Action Interlude

Write an acknowledgment to all parts of yourself either in this book or in your journal.

I, ____(fill in your name)____, am a spiritual being, a unique soul who uses my mind through resonating frequencies to animate my body into actions that produce the results I see around me. I have within my power the ability to use all parts of my being to create the results I desire.

Can you begin to see yourself in those terms?

manifestations in the physical realm. Awareness is the ability we have to recognize the effects of our actions on both the physical and nonphysical world.

What Your Mind Looks Like

Crossing this mental hurdle may take time. An image helps. That is what it took for me to embrace my mind in a way that skyrocketed my ability to use it more efficiently. Join me for a trip to our family farm in north Alabama, the summer of 1994.

It is ten years past my medical school graduation. As a practicing radiologist, I look at millions of images of different parts of the body: bones of the hands and feet, livers and spleens, lungs and hearts, brains and spines. The average number of exams each radiologist in my practice reads per year is 23,000. Exams range in image count from 1 to 1,000 pictures of the body. It is June, and in the evening calm, thousands of toads, frogs, and crickets perform with symphonic precision. June bugs bump against the kitchen window. I watch a praying mantis, still as a statue. My parents and I are visiting at the oak pedestal kitchen table, a focal point for farm activity. My father asks me one of the most pivotal questions of my life: "Lori, will you draw me a picture of the mind?"

"Sure," I confidently reply, and I draw a brain covered with squiggles that we in medicine pompously call a convolutional markings."

He states, "That looks like a brain. Can you draw a picture of the mind?"

I answer humbly after several minutes of contemplation. "No."

He then picks up a short golf-score pencil standing on its head and draws a picture of the mind and its relation to the body that was first drawn by Dr. Thurman G. Fleet.

The Stick Man

The image (Figure 1) consists of a large circle bisected into an upper and lower half and a smaller stick-like body dangling from the bottom. The upper half represents the conscious mind; the lower, the subconscious mind. The circle is larger than the body because the nonphysical self (spirit, mind and awareness) is much larger than what is encompassed by a physical being.

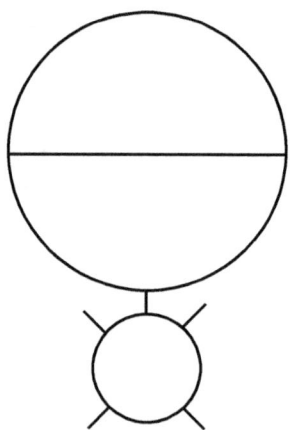

Figure 1. Artist's rendering of Dr. Thurman Fleet's idea popularized by teachers of Concept Therapy, Curtis Sliwa, Bob Proctor, and the Proctor Gallagher Institute.

My father had studied Bob Proctor's "The Born Rich Learning System" program. Daddy explained that the conscious mind is the thinking part of the mind that takes in information through our senses. It is also the place where we have the freedom to choose how we respond to information received. We can choose to accept, reject, or neglect any idea we give ourselves or receive from outside. The subconscious mind is the feeling part of the mind where emotions are generated and memories are stored. Subconscious readily accepts any idea turned over to it from the conscious mind. It stores those ideas in a filing system shaped by our paradigms. Feelings are resonations with either memories or hopes. These vibrations cause physical responses within and without our bodies.

Three Sources of Worry, Fear and Doubt

We just crossed a hurdle. Did you feel it? It feels more comfortable now to accept that we are more than our physical bodies. Next, recognize who exactly provides diseases with their trappings of worry, fear, and doubt. Just where do those illnesses "shop"? You already know the answer. It is fashion designed with more foresight, skill, and precision than Prada. We each provide the clothing that disease models. It shops in a storehouse of the subconscious mind. Our memories are stored in the subconscious mind. Our genetic programming, interaction with the world and our paradigms are three parts of the subconscious mind that empower disease.

Genetic Programming

Through humanity's collective consciousness, human beings have amassed a history with illness and disease going back to the beginning of time. Early human records provide evidence that diseases resulted in the sick being ostracized, impoverished, or slaughtered. Current human records indicate that in many parts of the world, this is still the case. Collective memories shape our societal thoughts and influence us as individuals through our genetic programming. Is it any wonder that when disease hits close to home, we begin to worry?

If you have ever grown pumpkins and placed a small one inside a can or other strangely shaped container as it is growing, the pumpkin will grow into the shape of the container. Rupert Sheldrake provides one cohesive theory that explains a similar process in fields of energy. This theory states that organizing energy fields exist around living beings (plants and animals) that carry the blueprints for the shape or morphology of the creature, even when it is in an embryonic state. For example, a salamander egg has a morphogenic field surrounding it that is the shape of the adult salamander. This field serves to organize random activity so that the resulting creature grows into the right shape and size and functions correctly. Dr. Sheldrake theorizes that through the process of morphic resonance, the information from the morphogenic field is communicated among members of the same species both locally and over distance. This theory helps to explain how our genetic programming shapes our perceptions and our lives. The morphogenic theory also helps to explain the role our environment plays in molding our thoughts.

Our Environment

Genetic programming is one source of uncharacteristic emotions that clothe illnesses; another source is our environment. We pick up on negative vibrations that radiate from other individuals suffering illness in doctors' offices, pharmacies, and hospitals. Consciously or unconsciously, we tune in to the negative emotions of overworked and underappreciated caregivers. When disease-treatment survival statistics and negative scientific results broadcast, we allow them into the subconscious mind without a conscious thought. These environmental sources feed fear with the same gusto that gasoline empowers a flame.

Memory Storage

Where else do uncharacteristic negative emotions come from? The most potent source is from the storehouse of memories that form our *worldview*, another of our paradigms. A current event resonates with a memory that feels similar, and, before we know it, we are trying to cope with the current situation using the same mechanisms we employed as a child.

My dear uncle asked me just a day before he died to examine his leg. He thought he might have a blood clot. I examined his leg, as did his wife, a registered nurse. His leg was warm and his pulses were strong. There was no unusual swelling or redness. No cord was palpable that is sometimes felt when a blood clot lodges in one of the major leg veins. My uncle died a day later from a blood clot. I was stunned and I wondered if I could have done something more to prevent this tragedy. I used all of my doctoring skills, yet he still died of the very thing he feared. Or perhaps he had an insight that a blood clot was affecting his body.

Strong memories are stored in our subconscious mind during times of shock, be it a happy or a grief-laden shock. Memories also can be stored by spaced repetition. To this day, whenever I am requested to examine the Doppler study of a person with suspected clot, a little voice inside says, "Lori, remember how it felt when Uncle Jerry died." If we do not take immediate action, then worry, fear, and doubt creep in, even though it is totally unfounded and irrational. That is how our paradigm works. We get into a situation that vibrates in harmony with an emotionally charged event from our past, and, unless we choose to steady our conscious mind, we will live out our lives using the same strategy that we applied during the initial crisis.

Reflect and Replace Your Negative Emotions

What is the appropriate response when these memories intrude on our current lives? Use self-talk to immediately reject the thought or to put the associated feelings and knee-jerk reactions in the rightful place in your history. For example, I might say to myself, "I acknowledge that I felt confused when Jerry died, and that memory of the past sharpens my focus on my current patient. Any other feelings about the past do not serve me now."

Most of these memories come from events that happened when we were very young. Any of the emotions attached to these events can be rekindled with vigorous intensity whenever you encounter a similar situation throughout your life. You may remember your grandmother afflicted with cancer. You may recall your grandfather groaning and unable to sleep. You may relive the shame of having an unsightly birthmark, or you may conjure odors associated with strong antiseptics used to clean up after a sick loved one.

My grandfather died of tuberculosis before antibiotics were discovered. At the time, my father was seven years old, his big sister was twelve, and his little brother was two.

To keep the rest of the family from contracting the disease, people used a popular disinfectant product with a distinctive odor to clean all surfaces in the home. If I held the bottle cap in from of your nose right now, you would be able to tell me exactly what product it is. What do you think happens every time my aunt, uncle, and father smell that disinfectant? Memories flood back of the prolonged illness and ultimate demise.

Sometimes though, we may be too young to retain a clear memory. Instead, a smell may simply conjure a feeling. It may cause a knot in the pit of the stomach or a wave of grief or a bout of confusion. That is how a current encounter with disease stirs up a quagmire of feelings from your past.

Worry, fear, and doubt are pervasive when illness enters our lives. We create a version of the disease in our mind that is as powerful as a conjured demon. Suave and seductive, it tempts us to fall back into thought patterns that counteract the abundance we desire and deserve. This is a natural part of our introduction to disease. If we don't know what it is, even more worry, fear, and doubt creep into our subconscious mind and create chaos that halts our normal existence. It is our job to recognize that illness is neither good nor bad; it simply is. We can learn to grow through the affliction just as skillfully as we can learn to grow through any other process that changes our lives.

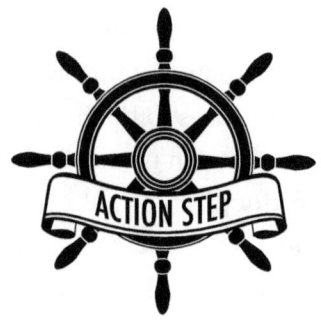

Reflect on your childhood, and recall any shocking events that created or continue to create feelings of worry, fear, and doubt. Search your memory for sensory triggers that cause you to revisit that memory. Write in your journal the name of the event, the trigger, and the prevailing emotion that is associated with that event. If there is more than one, write as many as your intuition tells you are important to write about.

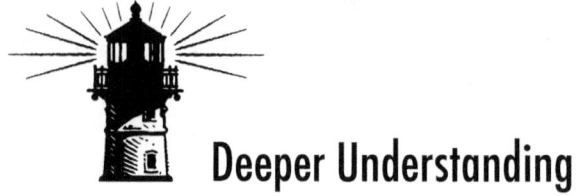

Deeper Understanding

Mere Christianity, C. S. Lewis, Harper Collins, New York, NY, 1952.

Dr. Thurman C. Fleet, Founder of "Concept Therapy": explore his work on- or off-line.

The Tipping Point, Malcolm Gladwell, Bay Back Books, Boston, MA, 2002.

Cells, Minds and Morphic Fields, Rupert Sheldrake and Bruce Lipton, A dialogue at Seattle, Washington, USA, August 2007 available as streaming audio on the internet.

The Born Rich Learning System by Bob Proctor is available at www.mindtamers.com, as are some of his other programs.

Chapter 3
Why Did I Do That?
(Cure the Unexplainable)

*A fanatic is one who can't change his mind
and won't change the subject.*
— Winston Churchill

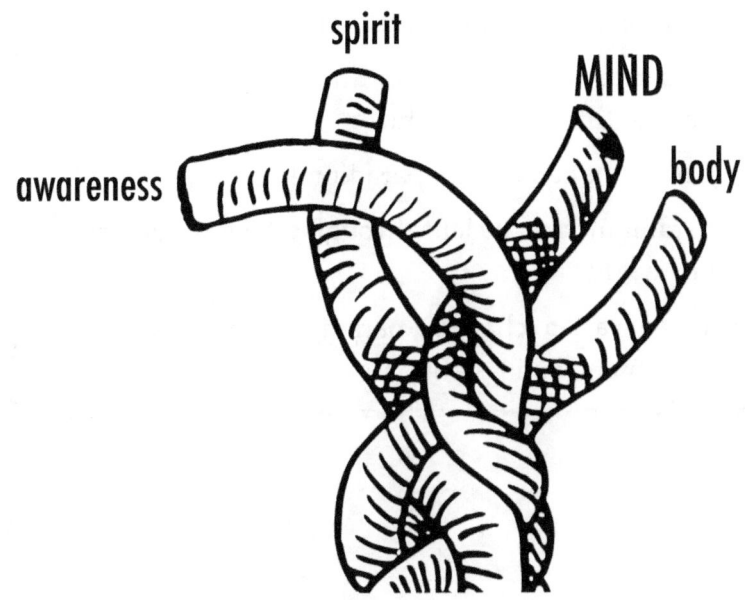

Lesson Summary

- Think of the mind in two parts: (1) conscious or thinking mind: accept, reject, neglect ideas; (2) subconscious or feeling mind: feeling, emotions, memories, cannot reject what you allow in.
- Subconscious mind does not know the difference between past, present, and future or between truth and fiction.
- Conscious intellectual faculties are not operational until about age six and then continue to develop up until about 25.
- Reinforcing the same idea over time forms habits.
- Habits are actions we take unconsciously; we don't have to think about them.
- Groups of habits form paradigms.
- Paradigms are the lens through which we observe our world.
- Three ways to change a paradigm are shock, agreement, and repetition.

Stan's Story

Stan slumps in the back seat of his mother's Suburban. They converse about the upcoming Scout trip with the brevity characteristic of parent-preteen conversations.

"Stan, did you finish all your homework this week?"

"Yes."

His mother relaxes. "Great! Then you'll have time to play with your friends before you pack for the camp out."

Stan lives for time with his neighborhood friends. He goes to a private school; they go to public. Stan loves being a Boy Scout; many of his friends are not. He cruises on his bike around the neighborhood and finds them. Mitch and the rest of the boys are lounging in the front yard at Pete's. After a brief discussion, they mount their bikes and whiz off to enjoy the whims that 12-year-old boys enjoy when they're not being rushed here and there for sporting events, school commitments, and music lessons.

Late Sunday night, Stan remembers some unfinished homework and sheepishly explains, "Mom, I did have math homework, and I left it at school."

"Stan, you lied about having homework, didn't you?"

Stan replies, "Yes."

His mother sighs, "Stan, why would you lie about a simple thing like homework? Why did you do that?"

Stan blurts, "Why? I don't know why! It just happened!"

No matter how many times his mother asks the question or even Stan asks the question of himself, he always get the same answer: "I don't know."

Why Did I Do That?

Are we any different as adults? Have you acted in a

certain way and then had no idea why you behaved in that manner? If you take the time to log your experiences and are mindful of the present, you will find you perform many actions and you have no idea why you do. This chapter is designed to answer that question once and for all.

Parents be warned! If your child reads this chapter, "I don't know" may be replaced with an answer that leaves you at a loss for words. This happened to me several years ago. At first it was a task to explore the reasons behind the answer to this question. Now it is easier. I challenge you to do the same as you walk through life and encounter people who do not know why they do the things they do.

Memories, Habits and Paradigms

Why we do the things we do is related to the relationship between our stored subconscious memories and the formation of our paradigms. Recall the discussion of the subconscious mind as the memory storehouse. While people oversimplify and believe we think in pictures and sounds, there are at least 12 languages of the mind.

Memories are stored as multifaceted vibrations that contain components of all of the mind's languages. This is partially explained in the theory of quantum holography. When the memory is recalled to the conscious mind—usually by current association with a similar image, sound, symbol, or smell—we resonate with the same emotions of the stored memory. The more times this memory is raised to the conscious level, the more it becomes engrained in our thinking pattern and eventually forms our paradigm. The paradigm is the way we see the world. It is the lens through which we experience our world. We look through this perspective, and what we see back is truly a reflection of our habits. Most great thinkers, philosophers, and scientists agree that the world is a relative experience based on our perception.

So what role does this have with regard to your health? Events that happen early in life can affect your health care decisions as an adult. If you did not like shots as a child, it is unlikely that you will look forward to a physician visit when you might get a shot as an adult. My mother and her siblings grew up at a time when the community nurse would come to their farm to administer vaccinations. One of my aunts hated shots so much, she would run and hide in the cotton patch until the nurse gave up and left. She managed to avoid almost all of her childhood vaccinations this way. She is still not a big fan of visiting nurses.

Children think very little about why they do the things they do. Before the age of six, it is almost as if the child is operating with only the subconscious mental faculties. The complex brain connections that allow understanding of abstract thought and reason have not yet developed in the brain. Every person goes through this phase of development and events that occur before we have the ability to limit what lodges in our memory become lodged deep in our subconscious mind. This means that everything in our lives is touched by our childhood environment and shaped by the people who were around us at that time. We hardly stop to realize what the effect these things might have on our personalities, likes and dislikes, and habits because we do not understand what shapes us when we are very young.

Habits are Unconscious Actions

The answer to Stan's question and to your question comes through a full understanding of the relationship between stored memories, the formation of your paradigm, and the role the paradigm plays as you experience similar situations in the present day as you continue the journey through life. All influences that shape your subconscious mind are stored as memories. Remember, mind is movement. The theory of quantum holography suggests that memory is a multifaceted vibration saved similar to a hologram.

This hologram-like vibration includes everything about the memory. It includes all of the sensory information you

Action Interlude

Keep a journal for one day of your actions as they relate to your body, physical fitness, and wellness. You might include what you eat, how you use your body, how it feels, if you have a visit to a health-care provider, what you say, or what you hear. The entries can be short. Include what the action is that you could capture with a camera or hear caught on a tape recorder, how you felt, what you did in response, and the reason you responded the way you did. Record action, feeling, response, and reason.

Next, after you keep this log for a day, review your written words, and recall Stan's story. If you ask yourself why you do the things you do, what is your answer? Are you really any different from Stan?

experienced at the time, usually with a vivid visual component as well as all emotions you felt. You have the ability to recall this memory to the conscious mind any time you are reminded of an event. Have you ever thought about the word *remind*? To remind is to bring back to the conscious mind again. So when you remind yourself, you are actually reaching into the subconscious mind and bringing to the level of consciousness a stored memory.

When the memory is recalled to the conscious mind, we experience the same emotions and set up the same vibration stored in the original memory. This vibration affects our actions, and our actions then affect our results. So Stan is not lying to his mother when he says he doesn't know why he did the things he did any more than we lie to ourselves. We simply fail to understand that when we act, often it is based on a mechanism that served us in a previous experience. For example, if you ran away and told the teacher when you were bullied at school, then in adulthood, when you feel you have been wronged in the workplace, you will tend to withdraw yourself from the situation and tell your supervisor. Those early protective responses that we learn shape our future reactions and behaviors.

Reinforcement Forms Habits and Paradigms

The more success we have with a certain strategy over time, the more likely we are to keep using that strategy. Eventually, these stored memories form our habits, and our habits over time form our paradigms. Our paradigms reflects the way we see the world. What we see outside of ourselves is a direct reflection of the habits and thoughts and feelings that form our attitude and that we have employed over time. That is a paradigm. Paradigms and memories are unique to each individual. Think of how differently you recall an event from another person who was also there and witnessed the same event. A paradigm can be a set of blinders that will not allow us to see anything but what is in harmony with our way of thinking.

Shift Your Paradigm Three Ways

Paradigms are shifted three ways. The fastest is through shock, the second is through agreement, and the third through willful intervention combined with spaced repetition of the new desirable paradigm. Willfulness for a particular outcome develops only when backed by passionate desire.

Shock

Stephen R. Covey tells of riding the subway and children run amuck all throughout the subway car. After looking around, it is easy to identify to whom they belong. Their dad stares out the window oblivious to the mayhem. Finally, Mr. Covey tells the gentleman, "Sir, your children are really disturbing a lot of people." The gentleman immediately returns to present and, bleary eyed, looks around. He absorbs the situation with his children pricking the other passengers and with this gentleman, Mr. Covey, talking to him. The dad replies, "Oh, you're right. I guess I should do something about it. We just came from the hospital where their mother died about an hour ago." Where Mr. Covey previously assumed the man was an irresponsible parent, this new information transformed him from dismay to understanding at seeing a fellow human being at one of the lowest points in life. That is an example of a paradigm shift through shock or surprise.

Another example of a paradigm shift caused by shock is related to unhealthy physical habits. My father-in-law, Gene Dent, casually smokes from the age of 14. His chest pains and breath shrinks when he walks the paths at Lakeland Community College, where he teaches in his late thirties. He sees his doctor and is treated for hiatal hernia. When a portion of the stomach slips into the chest where the esophagus is, it hurts and burns as reflux of stomach contents moves the wrong direction up the esophagus. He is referred to a surgeon for possible correction. After the initial consultation, a basic cardiac evaluation is advised before surgery. When test results come back, the doctor says, "Mr. Dent, you are going straight over to the Cleveland Clinic for coronary artery bypass surgery. Do not go home and get clothes. This is important."

In his hospital bed that night, he makes a promise to himself and throws away all of his cigarettes. Even though he tried to quit smoking on numerous occasions without success for 17 years, the shock of Death's bony elbow to his ribs removes all obstacles that previously kept him tethered to tobacco. He never craves nicotine and never smokes again.

It is very easy to shift your paradigm and drop the habit of smoking like a hot seat belt buckle when Death squeezes your hand. The subconscious mind is as alert as my father's comrades were when their ship was cowering in the path of the hurricaned tanker. Think of how long it takes to clear a path through a forest. With diligent repetitive work, it happens over time. Now think of how rapidly a tornado clears the forest. Shock works quickly in the forest of the subconscious mind where some of our beloved ideas are more vulnerable than the trailer parks that comprise the bulk of a tornado's diet.

Why Did I Do That?

Agreement

Whereas shock crashes into the subconscious mind, agreement slithers in through a side door. Agreement is another way paradigms are shifted, sometimes without our conscious realization that the process occurs. Agreement is a tactic often employed in sales and marketing. Savvy marketers understand that if they can get your agreement on at least three statements, you are unlikely to disagree on whatever is presented next in conversation.

We also use the tactic of agreement on ourselves when we begin to rationalize a position we would like to hold that the facts do not justify. Reflect on how your self-talk

Action Interlude

Take note of how often your subconscious mind is influenced by the agreement technique. Stop, look, and listen carefully the next time an advertising pitch catches your attention. See if the ad uses the premise of agreement before the call to action occurs.

Let's do something fun with salespeople on the phone. When you educate yourself through the experience, you decrease anxiety about being pitched. When you listen to someone who has refined sales skills, appreciate their talent and honestly compliment the salesperson on it. You can still say no to mal-aligned offers. Record these observations the next time you listen to a live pitch:

What hook did the salesperson use to catch my attention?

How many times did he/she encourage me to agree?

employs the agreement technique. Are you truly a savvy marketer who works in keeping with your objectives, or are you misaligned with your goals?

Diligent Cultivation of a New Idea

Finally, if you want to shift a paradigm without major life trauma or manipulation, then recognize how much your paradigm limits purposeful creation and collaboration. You can embrace so much more once you learn to shift you paradigms and notice how paradigms anchor others who still don't know why they make the same mistakes over and over. The intellectual faculty you exercise in this drill is the will. Will is the ability to focus on one thought for an extended period. The will is most effective when you have something worth fighting for in your life, like your health. Strengthen your will, and you will notice how much easier it is to leave unuseful paradigms in the past.

So why did Stan forget his homework, block it from his view, and then unconsciously lie about it? His weekend paradigm revolved around neighborhood friends and freedom. The homework became invisible to him because it was outside his paradigm. Many things become invisible because of our paradigms. This serves an important function because the volume of sensory information bombarding our conscious mind is far more than we can process. Paradigms help to protect us from sensory overload and mental malfunction. Paradigms are also the most common construction tools we use in creating our prisons to which Einstein referred. Strengthen your lifeline by identifying your paradigms.

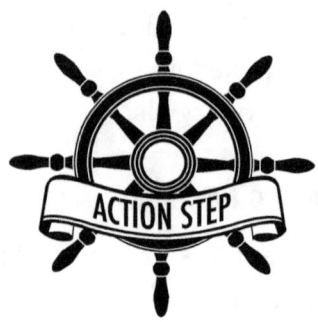

Pretend you are an undercover agent on an assignment, and use this exercise of will. When you arise in the morning, concentrate your thoughts on the two phrases: "Why did I do that?" and "Silly me." After a few moments of deep breathing and focusing of the will on the phrases, give yourself the suggestion that whenever either of the phrases is uttered within your hearing, you will hear it clearly, remember the context, and be able to recall the event later. When you are ready, proceed with your day. Make a mental note of the who, what, and why any time either phrase is spoken. In the evening, reflect upon what you have focused with your will. If you were the one who spoke the phrases the most, use this opportunity to remind yourself of how paradigms work in your life.

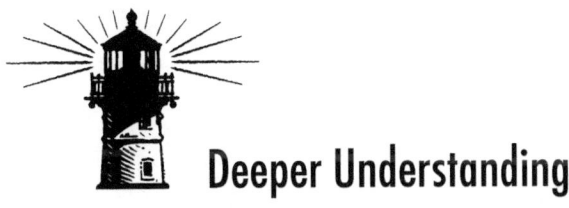

Deeper Understanding

Thought Particles: Building Blocks of Perceptual Reality; Binary Code of the Mind, Roy H. Williams, Wizard Academy Press, Buda, TX, 2001.

Essentials of Human Memory, Alan Baddeley, Psychology Press, East Sussex, Eng., 2005.

Twelve Languages of the Mind can be found at http://www.mondaymorningmemo.com/?ShowMe=ThisMemo&MemoID=1821

"Nature, Cognition and Quantum Physics" by Peter Marcer posted on the website of the British Computer Society. Dig even deeper on the internet and discover Marcer's ties to quantum holography, the idea of how memories are stored.

The Structure of Scientific Revolutions, Thomas Kuhn, University of Chicago Press, Chicago, IL, 1962.

The 7 Habits of Highly Effective People, Stephen R. Covey, Simon and Schuster, New York, NY, 1989.

Chapter 4
Where Did I Go?
(Find Your Purpose)

All the powers of the imagination combine in hypochondria.
—Mason Cooley

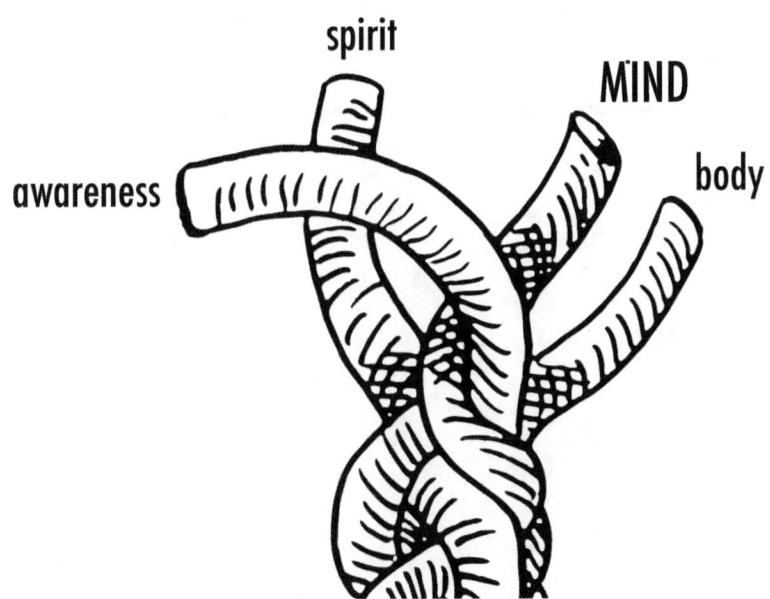

Lesson Summary

- Losing sight of or never finding your unique life's purpose leads to a short, unhappy lifespan.
- Stress is composed of good and bad, eustress and distress.
- Distress contributes to short lives and diseases.
- Recognizing and modifying our responses to stressors strengthens our vitality.
- The Ease-o-Stat™ is a tool to train you in recognition of your response to stress stimuli.

Don's Story

At one point Don was creative, productive, and deeply spiritual. Once he retired though, he made the mistake that many people do: he lost what he was fighting for. He gave up the thing that stimulated his mind during his entire working career.

Retirement creates time to relax and think. Unfortunately, Don became a slave to the will of others around him. He had uncommitted time; those around him were busy and had pressing items for him to do. Their task list for him related to their purpose. Don's life purpose got lost in the shuffle. His will withered from lack of use. Before long, he started feeling poorly. Don needed to see the doctor more frequently. In the United States, we have easy access to any doctor we choose and for whatever illness we want to discuss. In Don's case he wrapped himself up in a string of ailments that lasted the rest of his life. Don became a genuine hypochondriac. He had stomach ailments, muscle aches, bone pain, and headaches. Finally, he created a sleep disorder.

He lived to be 90 years old, but he worried himself away for the last 24.

Life Without Purpose Can Be Unhappy

If you lose sight of your life's purpose, your body gives you signs that you are out of balance. Your physical self tries to communicate that you are missing the point of life. Either we can choose to recognize the sign for what it is or we can truly believe that there's a problem with our body, and because we believe that, a problem soon develops that needs treatment. Don died a frail shell of the man who once lived, crumpled and distorted, unable to enjoy his last days because of the tremendous pain he had created. His body literally curled up. His face was drawn. It was as if the life had been sucked out of him. Everything he worried about did indeed happen. With his family supplying reinforcement, he was able to create many diseases for himself. Each one needed care and sometimes got better, but most of the time, they stacked upon each other until all you saw was illness when Don was near.

Action Interlude

Take a moment to write in your journal what *ease* means to you. Describe in detail how you feel when you are at ease.

Do not judge what comes out of your mind; just simply record it. Record it as word fragments, sentences, essays, or even as pictures. Depending on your current pathos, the emotions and feelings will come out of your mind onto paper in different ways. Remember, taking the time to write by hand has more of an impact on your subconscious mind than does recording the information in another form.

Next, do the same with the word *disease*. Take a moment to see what that word means currently to you. It may reflect experiences you've had with someone else in your life or personal experiences. See if you can take a moment to recognize any underlying emotions, which feed into your own dis-ease.

Stress

Have you ever really thought about the word *disease*, dis-ease? "Dis-" typically means abnormal or bad. "Ease" is the natural state our body longs for. If we are thinking actively and engaging ourselves in moving our lives toward a worthy goal, we are much less likely to be distracted by dis-ease. When we fill our hearts with stress, hatred, or jealousy, or engage in strife, we are much more likely to feel it in our body. This feeling is distress. The opposite of this is eustress. Eustress is felt after activities that recharge and revitalize us (Table 1).

Table 1. Physical Signs of Distress and Eustress

Measurement Parameter	Distress	Eustress
Blood Pressure	Increased	Decreased
Heart Rate	Fast, Variable	Slow, Steady
Skin	Cold, Moist	Warm, Dry
Alertness	Heightened, Flight or Fight	Varies
Bowel, Bladder	Nausea, Increased Urge, Decreased Digestion	Normal, Regular

What do current scientific investigations reveal about distress and our bodies? There are acute and chronic stressors, and these appear to have interwoven and cumulative effects with regard to some disease processes. Both stimuli cause harm when a negative emotional response is elicited. This leads to activation of the sympathetic nervous system and the hypothalamic/pituitary axis. It can be complicated by inadequate health maintenance.

Physiologic changes occur in the body and if not checked, can contribute to increased risk of physical and psychological disease. A few of the conditions stress contributes to are colds, depression, HIV/AIDS, slowed wound healing, infections, rheumatoid arthritis, asthma, and cardiovascular disease. Jobs that are perceived by the worker as hectic or highly demanding and that do not allow the worker individual decision-making opportunities and personal freedoms are environmental factors that over time lead to job-related stress, a form of distress. The purpose of this chapter is to study underlying emotions that lead people to these defining events that have a negative effect on their health. Let's start with ignorance versus knowledge.

Recognize Stress

Ignorance is a state of unawareness. When we recognize that we are ignorant of information, this causes worry and doubt in our conscious mind. Worry and doubt translate into fear in our subconscious mind. Fear that constantly plagues the subconscious mind is translated into anxiety in the body. We can become so conditioned to a state of anxiety that we fail to recognize it in our body. This is what is meant when someone asks you if you feel stressed. That person is really asking if you recognize signs of anxiety in your physical body on a conscious level. Ask yourself, "Do I feel distressed?" While there are many different levels of tolerance of stress, it is far more common for people to ignore signs of stress within the body that signify underlying fears, worries, and doubts than it is for them to have a high tolerance level for stress. Over time, especially if we are suppressing knowledge of stress and anxiety within our body, the result is depression and anger that is turned inward. Any strong negative emotion that is turned inward results in dis-ease and disintegration of the body.

> ## Action Interlude
>
> Review the physical signs of stress in Table 1. Ask yourself these two questions as you become more conscious of stress both as distress and eustress:
>
> **Is this a threat?**
>
> **Can I cope with it?**

Modify Your Stress Response

On the other hand, if you are in a state of awareness and continue to grow in awareness through knowledge and study, you develop understanding rather than ignorance. Understanding is a positive process in the conscious mind, which develops faith. Faith is the ability to believe in the incredible and to see the invisible and to receive the impossible. Strong faith develops a sense of well-being in the subconscious mind, a sense of self-assurance that cannot be found in any other way. This sense of well-being leads to expression of all emotions, positive and negative, rather than suppression, and this leads to a state of acceleration instead of depression because well-being vibrates at a higher frequency. It attracts everything necessary to move you forward toward your goals and life's purpose at a higher speed. This acceleration, as opposed to depression, creates a sense of being at ease because you are living proactively. This leads to relaxation and creativity, as opposed to disintegration. You choose to change your perception of the obstacles in life that used to cause you distress when you develop habits that condition you to look for opportunity and to avoid worry, fear, and doubt.

Train Yourself with the Ease-O-Stat™

The real key to freedom is faith based on understanding. How can you tell if you are at risk for disintegration or if you are moving toward acceleration and creativity and growth? One way is to use a measuring tool that helps you judge the

Action Interlude

See Appendix 1, and make yourself an Ease-o-Stat™. This tool is a measure of how you feel with regard to events in your life. Start each morning with your Ease-o-Stat™ at zero. Carry it with you so that as you go through the day, when an event happens, you can gauge your reaction to the event. If you have a strong positive reaction, move your Ease-o-Stat™ in the direction of the positive numbers, using the scale of one to ten to move forward. As you have positive reactions, keep adding to the positive score. If you have events that cause a negative reaction, move in the opposite direction, and take note of where you end up during the course of your day. Use this tool frequently until you develop the habit of recognizing consciously what your reaction is to certain stimuli. The Ease-o-Stat™ is only a temporary tool. Eventually, you will train your subconscious mind into the habit of gauging your response and know how you want to end your day. At the end of this chapter are conditions to determine where your Ease-o-Stat™ is currently set.

effects of external and internal influences on your ease or disease spectrum. I call this tool the Ease-o-Stat™. Think of the Ease-o-Stat™ as you would a thermostat. A thermostat is a cybernetic mechanism that controls a room's temperature. If external influences cause the room to become warm, the thermostat takes note of the change in the external influence and adjusts so that the temperature in the room is maintained at a very narrow margin of error. An Ease-o-Stat™ works in the same way.

Your goal will be to end your day with more feeling of ease rather than dis-ease. The first step is to recognize what ease feels like. The second step is to develop a standard for its measurement. There are many psychology tools that measure eustress and distress. Think of the Ease-o-Stat™ as an inverse of those tools. Although they offer an objective measure of stress and can be very useful for gathering data for research studies, that is not our goal. Our goal is to provide a personal tool that is specific for you. No two people experience ease the same way. This tool is designed to be customized to your current feelings and will change as your feelings change.

Your Unique Perspective

A big mistake individuals who are prone to a pattern of illness make is handing over their life's purpose to other people. You must recognize your unique place in this universe and find the reason you are here right now. Once you are on the path to this discovery, never lose sight of it, and never ever give it up to follow someone else's purpose. The ring of altruism is sweet and the result as bitter as a green persimmon. Every individual has his or her own purpose, and even though your purpose may resonate with the purpose of others, you must seek and maintain your unique ability to bear your own fruit in due season.

The absence of meaningful purpose leads to real physical symptoms. In other instances disease and chronic care-giving may cause you to lose sight of your life's purpose. Sometimes the habit of caring for others makes us invisible to ourselves.

Finding Purpose

If you feel lost, you must stop and discover or rediscover why you are here now. The secret to uncovering your life's purpose is first to determine what major paradigm forms your worldview. Ask yourself what underpins your philosophy of life, your outlook on how the world works. The paradigm may be science; it may be God; it may be humanism or something else. You as an acorn cannot fall far from the tree trunk of your oak. You perceive everything in life through the lens of your worldview. If you cannot see your purpose yet, then you may need to clean your lens, sharpen your focus, or perhaps have a lens transplant.

Next, you must be utterly convinced that your worldview is right for you. If you hold any doubts, you will need to continue with actions and activities that provide clarity around your choice for this important paradigm. Some activities that increase clarity in this regard include daily study of materials that help you find the truth about that paradigm; introspection to see if intuitively you have doubts about aspects of this topic; and discussions with others who are already very clear in this regard. If doubts remain after at least a year of dedicated study, then consider exploring another worldview.

Once you are clear about your worldview paradigm, it doesn't take long before you recognize how you can serve that cause effectively. Look for the activities that give you joy. Joy is a high-frequency emotion in which we resonate with others who are successfully carrying out their life's purpose. Instances of joy help to sustain our passion and build faith in our abilities. Happiness and joy are totally different. Happiness is a fleeting emotion and is often spontaneous. Joy may be spontaneous too, but it can be found consistently when you are performing tasks that move you toward a worthy goal.

If you lack joy or lay aside joy to tirelessly serve as a caregiver to another, you may kill yourself if you are not careful. Uncle Louis painted himself into a deadly corner in a very short time. He was always a handsome man and his wife a faithful companion. As my aunt aged, she became more and more in need of care. Eventually Louis' wife became bedridden. Louis wanted her to be comfortable at home, so he had a hospital bed delivered to their living room. She was as comfortable as any bedridden person could be, and he faithfully took care of her every need: meals, hygiene, toilet, and laundry. He got very little rest and became invisible to himself. Over time, Louis became consumed by his service to her. A few years later we visited them at home for the last time. He was a shell of his former self. He confided in me that he had fallen asleep outside in his truck for several hours, and this bothered him because he normally had no problem finding energy to farm and take care of his wife. Her condition had not changed substantially. Louis died from complications of pneumonia less than a week later. Did he notice that he was stressed? Not in time to save his life. Just as with Don, once his own life's purpose became invisible, he shriveled and died.

Assess Your Stress

This chapter introduces you to the idea of the Ease-o-Stat™ as a tool to help you gauge which direction you are moving in. Are you accelerating or are you disintegrating? The second law of thermodynamics discusses entropy. Electrons slow down. Moving objects slow down. Everything slows down. Energy must be added to the equation in order to move in the opposite direction. Once you know how to fully use your Ease-o-Stat™ and create awareness of ease and dis-ease within your subconscious mind, you will be able to know exactly when you need to add energy to your system to avoid long-term effects of fear and anxiety, otherwise known as disease.

If we nourish our will and the things that are really important to us, we will avoid the trap that led to years of misery for Don and others like him. This is another chance to stand up for yourself and tame your mind.

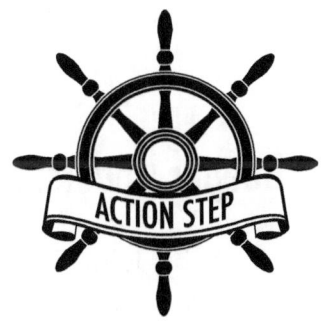

Stress Primer

Use your Ease-o-Stat™ to measure your personal response to the following stress stimuli. What is most important to you is how you feel or felt about the event in question.

Mourning after the loss of a loved one, human, animal, relationship, or job

Caregiving

Type of job (highly demanding and lack of personal freedom or control)

Natural disaster

Work or school difficulties

Victim of accident, robbery, law suit, rape, or assault

Arrest

Business readjustment

Marital or family stress

Lower socioeconomic status (real or perceived)

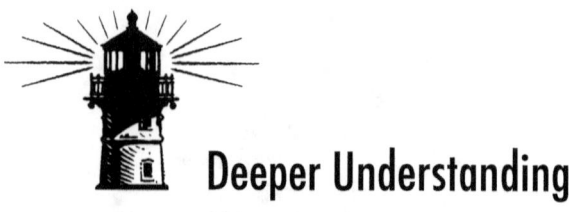

Deeper Understanding

The Mindbody Prescription, by John E. Sarno, M.D., Time Warner Book Group, New York, New York, 1998.

"Effect of Mindfulness-Based Stress Reduction on Immune Function, Quality of Life and Coping in Women Newly Diagnosed with Early Stage Breast Cancer," by Witek-Janusek et al., in *Brain, Behavior, and Immunity,* August, 2008.

"Socioeconomic Status, Antioxidant Micronutrients, and Correlates of Oxidative Damage: The Coronary Artery Risk Development in Young Adults Study," by Janicki-Deverts et al., in *Psychosomatic Medicine,* June 2009.

"Psychological Stress and Antibody Response to Influenza Vaccination: When Is the Critical Period for Stress, and How Does It Get Inside the Body?" by Miller et al., in *Psychosomatic Medicine,* March–April 2004.

Ease-O-Stat™ http://www.easeostat.com.

Chapter 5
Reset Your Ease-O-Stat™
(Nullify Stress)

The test of a first-rate intelligence is the ability to hold two opposed ideas in the mind at the same time, and still retain the ability to function.
—F. Scott Fitzgerald

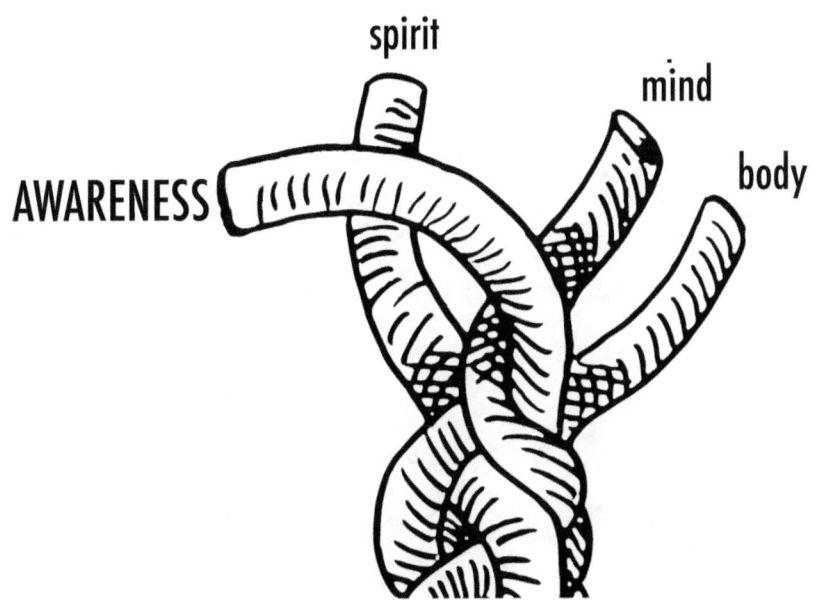

Lesson Summary

- Any long-term habit is not easily changed.
- You will have to introduce a new idea repeatedly for feelings of discomfort and/or terror to pass.
- You will tend to dismiss a new idea as a whim.
- Focus and fantasize on how you will feel once a new idea takes hold. How will you enjoy it?

Mary's Story

Not long ago, I met an amazing lady I will call Mary. She is beautiful and confident and carries herself with an uncommon air. She is aging with grace and has the means to enjoy her wisdom years. When she discovered I was a doctor, she volunteered, "I had a liver transplant." I was stunned. I have met many individuals who survived liver disease and subsequent transplantation, but never one who looked so radiant. When I shared that fact with her, she laughed and admitted that she spent a great deal of time very ill before transplantation. She was so sick for so long that she developed a special relationship with her gastroenterologist and his wife, Lisa. After many years, a transplant matched her, and her doctor called. At her next appointment, he disclosed a concern his wife had voiced on hearing the good news about the match. The wife said, "She has been sick for so long, do you think she knows how to be a well person?" He replied, "Lisa, she never learned how to be a sick person." As she heard the words from her doctor, she laughed and assured him she would be his best "well patient" if given the opportunity—and she is. Mary says, "I ask myself, 'Why am I the one that got to survive?'"

Action Interlude

Make a list of three things you want to enjoy doing with your body once you are acting well. If you haven't been acting well for a long time, this may be very uncomfortable. Do it anyway. Reflect on why this is uncomfortable.

The Joy of Discomfort

If someone were to ask you, Do you remember how to act well?" what would your answer be? Humans have the amazing capability of free choice, and we change our minds often. What this means is that we forget skills we set aside when they are not needed. Sometimes we must work hard to relearn neglected skills. Have you ever thought of acting well as a skill? Just look around in any public place. There are people of all ages. Some enjoy their walk through life; others believe their incarceration has been forced upon them from outside, but really the prison is of their own making.

Whatever state you operate in, acting sick or acting well, if you have acted that way for more than three months, it has become a habit. It is a comfortable state for you. Your subconscious mind develops a pattern of that way of acting and then carries out that pattern. If opportunity arises to change that pattern, as it did for Mary, it feels uncomfortable.

Long-term Habits Are Hard to Change

Imagine that your subconscious mind is a factory creating a product we will label S for sickness. The reinforcement that you are sick, your disease tattoo, comes from your own thoughts, feedback from your environment, and through communication with others. Your conscious mind is like the supervisor at the plant. It passes the template, the S ideas into the assembly line and makes sure all workers understand the product to be made: S. The subconscious mind uses all the resources it can attract from within you and from the rest of your world to create the product you ordered: S. It is an efficient factory; you get out more of what you put in.

One day your conscious mind inspires you to act well. Let's call that idea a W idea. It tentatively sends the W template, the idea down to the subconscious factory, and because the entire subconscious mind is working on the S-idea template to create more S for you, the W is rejected because the supervisor did not prepare the workers for a change. You pass the idea off as a whim because you misuse your intellectual faculty of reason. "Who am I to think about being pain free?" Your subconscious is trying to protect you from going in a direction you have not traveled for a long time. Consider it your quality assurance division at the factory. It recognizes a W idea out of step with the established S pattern and rejects it.

When management wants one thing and the workers produce something else, it causes discomfort. There are layoffs; people quit; there may be reassignments. The supervisor himself may be fired for not communicating effectively with the production line employees. Likewise, a W idea that enters the subconscious mind busy with the production of S from a template of longstanding S ideas feels just as uncomfortable. It takes time and reinforcement of the W idea before the production team in the subconscious mind feels comfortable about producing W results in your life.

The exact opposite is true, as well. If you are healthy and have a subconscious mind full of W ideas happily producing W, you act well and enjoy yourself. If there is a sudden overwhelming load of S ideas passed down into the subconscious—perhaps you are in an automobile accident and are suddenly paralyzed—your mind as well as your body feels uncomfortable. All of those factory workers want to reject the S they have not been trained to produce.

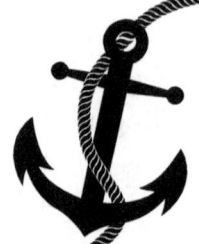

Action Interlude

Prescription for Changing Your Ease-o-Stat™

1. Use your Ease-o-Stat™ often until you are able to get a reading on yourself without looking at it. If this sounds hard, think about the skills you use to gauge other measurable factors. Are you able to tell when a loved one has a fever without using a thermometer? Are you able to tell if you are driving too fast without looking at your speedometer? Are you able to tell if a room is too hot without looking at the thermostat? If you can do any of these, you can learn to gauge your level of ease independent of the Ease-o-Stat™.

2. Make a list of ways you know you are in ease and a list of ways you know you are in dis-ease. These may include the rapidity of your breathing, the way you hold your jaw, or the carriage of your shoulders. Expand and contract these lists as you notice other signs of ease or dis-ease.

3. Begin to notice what activities leave you distressed and which ones leave you rejuvenated. Make a list of ten activities that refresh you and rank them from one to ten, with ten being the most effective at restoring your spirit.

4. As you find yourself feeling distressed or dis-eased, take a few minutes to use one of the activities you listed in Step 3, and refresh yourself. Repeat this for as long as necessary to notice a change in your vibration or in how you feel.

Focus and Fantasize

The bottom line is that, whether you transition from health into disease or from disease into health, either way will produce nonphysical and physical discomfort. You will be scared. The simple (but never easy) cure is to force yourself to do it even when you are afraid. Even if the idea terrifies, approach your terror and feed your subconscious mind ideas that move you toward the Ease-o-Stat™ setting you desire.

Imagine a chronic illness that lasts ten years. It takes an inordinate amount of energy just to think about active roles for self-care and care of others rather than focus on rest and death. The thought of expending all that energy terrifies. "Where will I find the energy?" "Will people trust me to do this for them after so long?" These questions enter the conscious mind.

Even though Mary strongly desired to be well again and mastered being well again by the time I met her, wellness mastery after disease comes only from a series of terrifying steps and breakthroughs after repeatedly resetting your Ease-o-Stat™. She worked very hard nonphysically, with her spirit, mind and awareness before she worked physically to see herself in perfect health. You can, too.

Let's reset the Ease-o-Stat™. The first step is falling in love with the idea of the benefits you'll enjoy from a new Ease-o-Stat™ setting. You must fall in love with the idea of how it will feel when you are well. Has your current condition kept you from certain activities? How will it feel to enjoy those activities again? When one falls in love, one often writes love letters. Write to yourself about the way you feel and what you do with your newfound energy and hope. Read and reread what you write multiple times a day. Record your writing in your voice and listen to it. Fantasize about it. Fall in love with this new W idea.

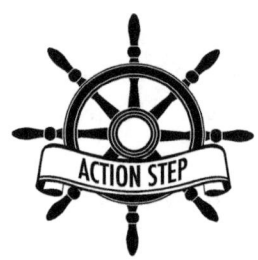

Read about Stella Adler on Wikipedia, and pay attention to what was unique about her teaching style. Which intellectual faculty did she ask actors to rely on during their performances?

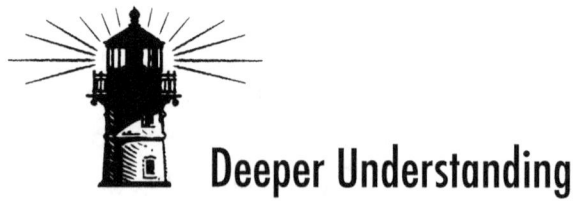

Deeper Understanding

The Art of Acting, Stella Adler, Applause Theatre & Cinema Book Publishers, New York, NY, 2000.

Psycho-cybernetics, by Maxwell Maltz, Pocket Books, New York, NY, 1969.

The Brain That Changes Itself, by Norman Doidge, M.D., Viking Penguin, New York, NY 2007.

Chapter 6
The Dance with Disease
(Face Illness without Fear)

The American child is a highly intelligent human being—characteristically sensitive, humorous, open-minded, eager to learn, and has a strong sense of excitement, energy, and healthy curiosity about the world in which he lives. Lucky indeed is the grown-up who manages to carry these same characteristics into adult life. It usually makes for a happy and successful individual.
—Walt Disney

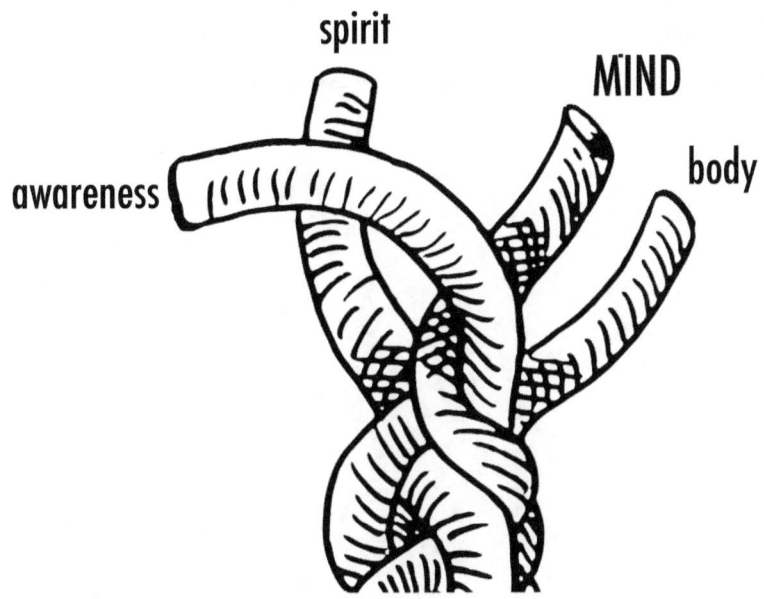

Lesson Summary

- Your imagination choreographs your dance with disease.
- You became an expert in imagining before you were six years old.
- Create a workshop for your mind, your "imaginasium," a place where you work out with your mental muscles.
- Universal laws define human existence. Work with them.

Sabrina's Story

It is May in New Orleans, sultry and fragrant. A line of young people dressed in caps and gowns twitches like the tail of an angry cat as the students await their turn on stage. One young lady is particularly grateful and proves to be a remarkable achiever. Sabrina graduates from high school as valedictorian, a tall, beautiful blond who plans a career in medicine. This is not the most remarkable of Sabrina's accomplishments. While other little girls learn tap, jazz, and ballet, Sabrina masters the dance with disease.

Fifteen years earlier, when Sabrina was three, her family received a dreadful shock. Sabrina's body was afflicted with cancer. Sabrina was young enough that she avoided the preconceived notions her family held concerning a cancer diagnosis. Notions like:

- This is so unfair!
- What did I do to deserve this?
- What can be worse than cancer as a child?

Cancer recovery to this three-year-old was no more onerous than corrective shoes. It was simply a part of growing up for Sabrina.

Every week, little girls all around New Orleans go to small dance studios where aging matriarchs pass on their knowledge of graceful carriage. Instead, Sabrina went to the hospital just as regularly. She learned the same lesson of graceful carriage with an uncommon depth because cancer is an uncommon dance partner for a child of this age. She lived near a children's hospital staffed with great specialists and stayed at home during therapy. Toxic medicines, intravenous lines, boring periods of sitting and lying around were just a fraction of the cost demanded of Sabrina and her family for her chance at a cure. Months of treatment became years, and Sabrina became physically frail.

Mentally and spiritually she remained stronger than ever. Even though she was extremely ill, Sabrina was aware that the nonphysical part of her being was where the dance began. She went to church and to school anytime she could. She was encouraged to grow in ways that the average child is not because her time on earth was perceived as shorter than most, and the results seemed miraculous. As a result, she encouraged other children to think differently about themselves. Perhaps the most inspiring feature about Sabrina and her growth was her gratitude. While Sabrina enjoyed every piece of life she was given, she never failed to thank God, and she showed her appreciation to those around her. Her hope beckoned to all who had the happy chance to interact with her as she grew. Seeing Sabrina enjoy her life proved even more beautiful than watching the fluid movement of any world-class dance master.

Action Interlude

Watch a performance of a dance company, an acrobat troupe, gymnast, figure skater, or a classic film star known for dancing. People and troupes particularly useful for the exercise are Gene Kelly, Ginger Rogers, Ben Vereen, Mikhail Baryshnikov, Cirque de Soleil, Stomp, and Martha Graham. Closely observe the performers in motion, and make yourself aware of your emotions as you watch. Write down observations as they come to mind.

A day came when her grateful parents announced guardedly to all that Sabrina's cancer was in remission. It continues to be so 15 years later at her graduation. Did Sabrina's grateful attitude, zeal for achievement, and fearless approach to recovery make the difference? Was it her discipline with regard to the inward motion of her body as she mastered the dance with cancer?

The Secret of Skill Mastery

Dancing is a physical skill similar to skiing. You've heard the occasional skier say, "I didn't learn to ski until I was an adult. Then I had to overcome my fear of going down a mountain." Ask them about their children and they say, "I enrolled my son in ski school when he was three. He had and still has no fear of any color run. He enjoys skiing so much more than I ever will." Children who learn to dance when very young are not self-conscious when they dance at their wedding or even on stage. They grow up dancing and do not consider the physical demonstration of the mastery they have over that aspect of their bodies something to get emotionally worked up about. Isn't that really the secret to mastering a new skill? Do it while you are young before you develop a self-fulfilling paradigm that tells you how difficult it will be.

The mastery of illness during childhood is no different. My medical subspecialty is in pediatric radiology, and people often ask me why. My reason is rather selfish: I prefer to work with children, who are usually not to blame for the circumstances of their illnesses and who heal with such grace that it reminds me to be grateful for every blessing. Really now, who am I to get upset about the cat missing the litter box when I have just met the most remarkable family with a very sick and yet very joyful child? So how do we as adults learn from these children with disease? How do we suspend our own fears about disease long enough to grow and master our bodies in this respect?

A Lesson From a Master

Take a lesson from a master. Perhaps the easiest way to do this is to begin by taking appropriate lessons, just as any student who desires to master a physical skill. We are looking for a master at engaging the adult mind in childlike wonder. There is no dispute that the absolute master of this skill in the past century was Walt Disney. During a period of realism in theater and on screen, Disney came up with a unique idea, to create animated pieces that would capture the dreams of children and adults. When that worked, he had unique ideas about building whole parks where families could come and remember the wonder of their youth. His legacy is the closest thing any living person will have to meeting Peter Pan or Mary Poppins. Isn't that the secret of real magic? Magic is any time we recognize the unlimited nature of human potential and its tie to the Infinite.

Walt Disney created a formula that allows individuals to suspend their current paradigms and to experience childlike wonder without repercussions from the rest of humanity. What are the basic components of this formula? Consider the process Disney called "imagineering." He chose a story to which many people could relate but that few Americans had personally experienced. He created in his imagination a vision of his customers feeling the impact of the story that would exceed any possible expectations.

Action Interlude

Listen to a song with lyrics that celebrate the freedom of imagination, for example, "Pure Imagination" from the original *Willie Wonka and the Chocolate Factory* movie or "The Age of Not Believing" from *Bedknobs and Broomsticks*.

Make a list of what is holding you back from exploring your imagination with the freedom you used to as a child.

He created a mastermind group of highly imaginative individuals with specialized knowledge in communication, engineering, animation, and design. These imagineers brainstormed his initial idea and devised ways to make his idea possible. They created an execution plan for the idea that included storyboards, a timeline, and where in Disney's grand plan this idea fit. The group would meet regularly until the idea materialized.

Once the movie launches or the ride opens, audience reaction gauges the imagineer's success. Audience feedback contributes to the success of future endeavors. Disney said, "Somehow I can't believe there are any heights that can't be scaled by a man who knows the secret of making dreams come true. This special secret, it seems to me, can be summarized in four Cs. They are Curiosity, Confidence, Courage, and Constancy—and the greatest of these is Confidence. When you believe a thing, believe it all the way, implicitly and unquestionably. When you're curious, you find lots of interesting things to do, and one thing it takes to accomplish something is courage."

Disney created the imagineering formula and taught it to his protégées so that even after his death, millions continue in delight as if Disney were still alive.

Disney described adults with a children's approach to life as "not afraid to be delighted with simple pleasures" and having "a degree of contentment with what life has brought."

Action Interlude

Ask yourself, "Can and will I think with the same wonder and freedom of a child any time I choose and thus achieve physical mastery over my body at an accelerated pace?" That is what Sabrina did and what millions of sick children teach themselves to do every year.

Create Your Imaginasium

Regain this ability as you recognize all parts of your personality, and permit each part to play its own role in your healing. This is best accomplished with full engagement of your imagination. Take the time to create a place in your mind you can visit that gives you comfort. It may be a palatial estate, a beach hut, a cottage in the woods, or other space that feels comfortable to you. Create the outside of your place of comfort and all the details about the inside of this place. Give it as many inner spaces and rooms as you need to accomplish daily imagination work within your life. If you are business-oriented, it could look like a corporate office with individual offices for the different facets of your personality and different production facilities for your activities. For a youngster, it might look like a tall sailing ship or a fantasy castle. Most important, you must invest enough of your preferences in the place, enough details to spark a desire to visit it every day. Begin visiting your place daily, and explore what it offers.

This is your "imaginasium," a place where anything is possible and can be enjoyed. Inside your space enjoy using your perfect body in ways you haven't been recently enjoying it. Perhaps it is a formal masked ball where you are able to dance without being self-conscious and you enjoy wearing those three-inch stiletto heels that look perfect with your ball gown. Your feet don't get tired here. The more you visit this workshop of the mind, the more you will be able to find facets of your personality buried there. The critical piece for this lesson is well described by Disney:

"I do not make films primarily for children. I make them for the child in all of us, whether we are six or sixty. Call the child 'innocence.' The worst of us is not without innocence, although buried deeply it might be. In my work I try to reach and speak to that innocence, showing it the fun and joy of living; showing it that laughter is healthy; showing it that the human species, although happily ridiculous at times, is still reaching for the stars."

Discover your innocence as you explore your inner space created for your own comfort.

The more time you spend dusting off the intellectual tools at your command that you put away when you left childhood, the more likely you will master your dance with disease. Remember that your imagination shrivels without use, and it will be uncomfortable getting into a habit of using it daily. Work through this discomfort until the new habit is formed.

You Are Already the Expert

Tempted to believe that Disney is the one of only a handful of true masters of imagination? On the contrary, you are already an expert at the use of imagination. Malcolm Gladwell discounts that idea with his concept of the critical amount of time it takes to become an expert in playing a musical instrument.

Repeated research demonstrates that the critical amount of time is 10,000 hours of focused practice with clear intention to improve. Now, review your own childhood. Were you intent upon using your imagination to explore your new world for the first five years of your life for all of your waking hours? Did you have difficulty separating reality from fantasy for those first five years? Let's say the average child under the age of five is awake and stimulated for ten hours a day. It would take only 1,000 days to become an expert at the use of the imagination. That is under three years. Now most children have the luxury of spending the majority of their time exercising their imagination until they start elementary school at the age of five or six. Even if they spend only six hours a day, they still become experts in use of the imagination in less than five years. Don't you qualify as an expert based upon hours you devoted to focused imaginative play as a child? If not, just how many hours of practice do you lack?

Your imagination is one of the most important intellectual faculties you exercise to change your habits and paradigms. Remember the three ways to change a paradigm: shock, agreement, and spaced repetition. Employ your entire imagination, and it becomes a safe environment for your subconscious mind to enjoy the fruits of change. It allows the protective portion of your personality, the one that hates change, to take a mini-vacation as you explore how it feels once the new idea is firmly accepted and becomes a habit. Your imagination is a time machine. It takes you to the future where you already enjoy the rewards of your labors.

Working with the Universal Laws

We are taught that the imagination is only a place to waste time on dreams that can never come true. That is a lie! Consider that every physical object in the world is the result of the creative use of the imagination without bounds. Great inventions—such as animated cartoons, Disneyland, the airplane, the car, and the light bulb—all originated in minds of individuals who would not accept their current reality as the limits of what is possible. If you think this does not apply to the health and longevity of your body, reconsider. This is what the world is all about. An idea backed by faith, an orderly plan, and enough energy applied to the plan must physically manifest in this world. This is a universal law. It is not the only universal law, and when you work in harmony with all of the laws, you will be amazed at what you are able to influence.

Take a moment and suspend your disbelief about the last paragraph. All of the great achievers throughout the ages recognized this one important concept and used it to achieve their life's work. If you are not taking advantage of the important gift of imagination, just try it for one month. You will soon discover that you have more of a role to play in determining your outcome that you ever imagined previously.

Why is this? We have surrounded ourselves with individuals who operate on the premise that the current results present in our lives, including our health, are a reflection of our potential. Even if we wanted to believe differently, until we learn to disregard thoughts that are not in keeping with our life's purpose, we will continue to be limited by the prevailing thoughts dominating the media, our work, and our home environment.

Once you recognize the freedom of thought you possess, you will never allow other individuals to determine your outcome again. You will take an active role in creating the outcome you envision in your imagination. It is at this point that you become the dance master, and disease must follow your steps. This is exactly what Sabrina accomplished with regard to her cancer. Not surprisingly, she sees no limits to what she can achieve in other realms of her life.

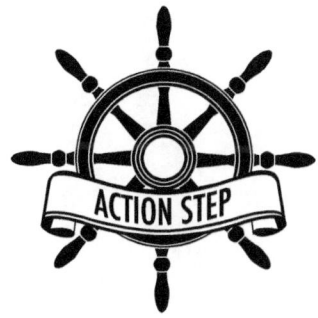

Spend at least five minutes per day for the next week working on the following details about your imaginasium, and write them in your journal.

What kind of path takes you there? How does it feel? What kind of dwelling is it?

Identify at least three rooms, what they look, smell, sound, and feel like. Determine how you will use these rooms.

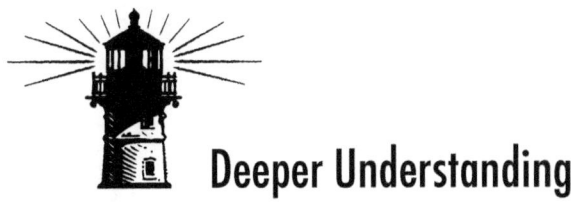

Deeper Understanding

Explore the whole-brain teaching approach of Donna Cercone, a gifted teacher and trainer, available at http://www.cerconelearning.com. (Donna Cercone's "Learning Room Story" from *Mega Learning* was the stimulus for the exercises in this chapter.)

Outliers, by Malcolm Gladwell, Little, Brown and Company, New York, NY, 2008.

Working with the Law, by Raymond Holliwell, DeVorss & Company, Camarillo, CA, 1939.

Chapter 7
From Mission Impossible to Mission Accomplished (Kindle Passion)

Do what you can with what you have where you are.
—Theodore Roosevelt

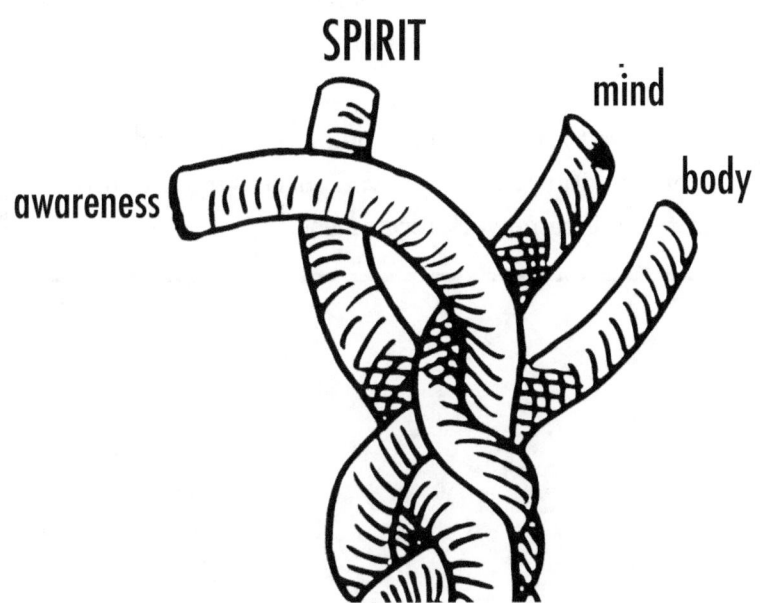

Lesson Summary

- Passion is the fuel that feeds the vehicle you are driving on your road through life.

- Practice your passion to recognize when an idea incites enough passion in you to fuel you into action.

- The vehicle driven by passion is a framework made up of your commitments, actions, associations, and mastery. It can be a push-pedal car or a racecar; you build it through your actions, failures, triumphs, and experiences.

- A desire to pursue a goal outside of areas where you previously have enjoyed success may require a different framework for success.

Jerry's Story

"Jerry is a different baby," his mother says to her oldest daughter. He wants water instead of milk. As a toddler, Jerry enjoys drinking large amounts of water, and this soon becomes an insatiable urge. All during childhood, he is thin and gains weight only when he approaches puberty. He gains weight in his trunk, skinny legs, and a wide midsection. He injures his hip, and for the remainder of his life walks with the characteristic limp of someone who has one leg shorter than the other. With skinny legs, a limp and the wide midsection, he looks like a chicken that almost made it across the road. Just as with Sabrina, Jerry's funny walk and water-drinking habits do not stand in the way of his love of life. Jerry develops a charismatic personality and is a fun-loving character. He becomes an engaging storyteller at a young age. Diabetes runs in the family, and his mother continually questions the family doctor about his water drinking and weight gain. The doctors tell him he is borderline diabetic, and he sometimes diets.

Jerry insists he wants to preach. After high school, he moves to a college several hundred miles away. He misses his spiritual and physical families so much that after one year, he transfers back home. He drives a school bus to earn money for his ministerial education. Both the children and their parents love Jerry. He woos and marries a bride with an equal amount of charisma and continues to study and grow. He is happy at home in Florence, Alabama, and after he graduates, he feels the desire to become a missionary. Rather than travel halfway around the world, Jerry seeks the spiritually malnourished individuals in the coastal United States. He and his wife move to LaRose, Louisiana, to minister to a small congregation that triples in size after his arrival.

On September 15, 1978, Jerry begins to have trouble seeing. The eye doctor sends him to another doctor, who admits him to the hospital in New Orleans. Although he is young, the symptoms indicate stroke. Before the doctors sort out his confusing medical history and his current complaint, he has a second stroke that affects all of his bodily functions. He is in intensive care for weeks. Finally, with a detailed medical history, doctors discover that Jerry suffered the majority of his life with both congenital diabetes mellitus and diabetes insipidus. While the doctors finally know how to treat him, they cannot reverse the organ damage from the two strokes. His kidney function is reduced. He must go on dialysis.

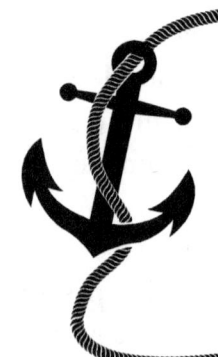

Action Interlude

Name your passion.

What is holding you back from relentless pursuit like Jerry's?

Because Jerry danced with disease all of his life, even without a conscious awareness, peritoneal dialysis becomes a way of life and a blessing. After six months of hospitalization, on March 31, 1979, he returns to LaRose. On the first Sunday in May 1979, he again preaches to his congregation and does so for the next ten years.

As his health declines, he and his wife move back to Florence, Alabama, and to the comfort of his origins.

Confined to a wheelchair, he entertains those who love him with witty stories and candid observations. Always tenderhearted, Jerry is the one who suffers the most when his mother dies. He dies two days later from a blood clot, an unexpected and relatively painless end to many years of chronic illness and hardship that most would have considered unbearable.

Passion Is the Fuel

Why is it that Jerry never viewed his illness as detrimental to his dreams? He had an all-consuming passion for preaching the Gospel. It was his strongest core desire; it fueled him with all of the energy the universe has to offer. Do you have anything in your life you are that passionate about? Is passion really that important anyway?

Passion is an emotion that we can imagine as fuel. It can fire all your heart's desires or all your fears and negative

Action Interlude

Recreate in your imaginasium the memory of your most passionate experience in each area below. Rate your passion intensity on a scale from 1 to 99, with 99 being the most intense.

Spiritual
Sport or physical activity
Intimate relationships
Family
Creative
Professional
Service

feelings. Passion is critical if you want to overcome obstacles that appear to be limiting your vitality. Nothing can replace the raw power of passion, or burning desire, in your role as a co-creator of your world. You must then use that energy to make a commitment, follow through with action, gather your forces, and master the task regardless of the obstacles. These actions are a framework for your success. Together, they make up the vehicle that you drive on the road of life, but if passion is not fueling your tank, you won't travel far.

When you get busy with day-to-day activity, you lose sight of the people, activities, and actions that incite passion. If it is difficult to remember how it feels to be wildly in love with a person, place, or activity, then it is time to reconnect with this powerful force at your command.

Rekindling these memories helps your body remember the feelings of passion that you experienced in those moments. This in turn will help you to recall that feeling and learn to associate it with some of your current desires. You may discover that you have lived a dispassionate life. Not to worry; the steps below will guide you into increased intensity.

Practice Passion Daily

You must practice passion often enough in your daily life that you become able to recognize when an idea fires you into action. Once you reach this stage, it is easier to reframe tasks that do not incite passion so that you see them through your passion. For example, no one is excited about going to the gas station and filling up the tank. People are excited about taking a vacation in the car, and, because filling up the tank brings them one step closer to the vacation, they can view that task through passion for their vacation.

Action Interlude

Pick one or two of these. If you are rereading this chapter, pick one you haven't tried before.

- Read the book of Mark from the Bible.
- Read a biography on Napoleon.
- Read Carol Burnett's autobiography.
- Watch several episodes from the first season of the television program Dallas.
- Reflect on the similarities of your own life with the life of one of these passionate individuals. What do you think makes the difference?

Refine and Store Passion

Do you have a framework for activity, a vehicle that is fueled by passion? Your ability to create is fueled by passion. Whether you have been using your framework is a different matter. Is your passion refined so that it is in a form you can use it? Is it readily available to you whenever you desire? All forms of fuel must be refined before they are compatible with different engines. Raw passion is useless unless it is refined into a form that serves your vehicle, your framework for worthwhile activity. It would also be an advantage to have a reserve store of passion handy when you really need to overcome major obstacles.

Let's examine the process of refining and storing your passion so that it serves you whenever you need it. Consider the lives of some passionate individuals: Jesus the Christ, Napoleon, Carol Burnett. Or, just to add one more to this eclectic collection, perhaps you would prefer to consider a fictional character that ties in nicely with the fuel analogy: J. R. Ewing, one of the main characters in the 1980s TV drama, *Dallas*. When you dig into the stories of these individuals, it becomes clear that these people are not passionate about just one thing. These passionate people focus the intensity of that passion on their dreams. They refine their passion. As you engage in this action interlude, be aware of what that laser-like focus allowed these individuals to accomplish.

If you find an unexpectedly large gap between what you perceive about their lives and your own, take immediate action. Start exploring ways to increase your awareness of your feelings. As you begin you may find that you are quite numb about most things. This is a common pattern in repressed households and is documented to contribute to disease manifestation. Keep right on gauging your feelings on a scale from 1 to 99 until the habit becomes automatic. This will take a minimum of 21 days and more than 1,000 repetitions. Somewhere along the way, you will begin to notice that some things do incite a stirring of passion when you engage in them. With more practice, you will find that just thinking about the activity elicits the same feelings that the actual activity does. If you spend enough time practicing, you can achieve the same intensity of feelings with regard to passion or any other emotion you choose with the pure use of your imagination. This is exactly the process good actors employ. They make it look easy because of the length and intensity of their practice.

Intense comic genius is a tribute to the amount of time actors discipline themselves and how freely they apply their imagination. They seethe passion by their excellent and spontaneous performances. To perform excellent improvisation takes an inordinate amount of practice at being funny and thinking on one's feet. This is an example of refining passion. As you begin to consider the champions in the area of your passion, examine their habits with the intent of identifying the way they constantly refine their passion.

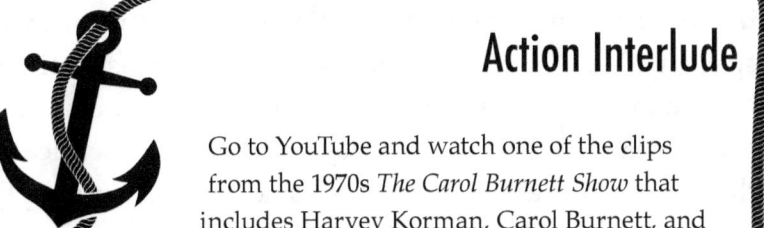

Action Interlude

Go to YouTube and watch one of the clips from the 1970s *The Carol Burnett Show* that includes Harvey Korman, Carol Burnett, and Tim Conway.

Passion Fuels Your Life's Framework

Passion provides the fuel, and appropriate action must accompany that passion if anything meaningful is to come of it. You cannot fill up your car's gas tank and expect it to take you somewhere if you are not willing to push the accelerator. The first step is to decide where you want your passion to take you, just like Jerry, who decided on preaching. Then you must plan and act to move in that direction. This requires cultivation of a habit of commitment. It means doing what you love when you are tired, hungry, and thirsty. Make a habit of getting passionate about how it feels to already have the results you desire, and you will find yourself totally committed to your goal. This is exactly how Jerry returned to his congregation in LaRose after his grave illness.

Jerry took advantage of another time-tested idea to move toward his vitality goal. He created a mastermind group. He had a team of doctors, nurses, family, spiritual mentors, and home-health professionals with whom he met regularly. He let them know exactly how he wanted to live. As you begin to see your unlimited potential regardless of the condition of your present health, you will need to assemble a team of experts to help you plan each step toward your goal. Select individuals you truly admire, who are successful in their specialty. Make a plan of how you will compensate these individuals for their service. Compensation does not necessarily mean money. Look for ways you can be of service to them. Return the favor; endorse someone else; and apply your skill set to his or her objective. Begin meeting with them regularly. After a certain level of rapport is established, these individuals will help you organize your plan for success and help you implement it. As you establish this habit, you will be amazed at the added depth of passion you are able to maintain for your goal.

Be Ready to Upgrade Your Vehicle

Follow your plan that is devised with the help of your experts. If it fails, make a new plan and keep driving. When logical steps toward a goal are followed and when you eagerly anticipate the revealing of the next few logical steps, a pattern of mastery emerges. Mastery is the ability to give yourself a command and to follow through. The achievement of mastery is the point at which you know you will never run out of passion to fuel your creative engine. Your only question at that point will be if the vehicle you are driving, the framework you have successfully used to move down this road, is robust enough to take your life where you want to go next.

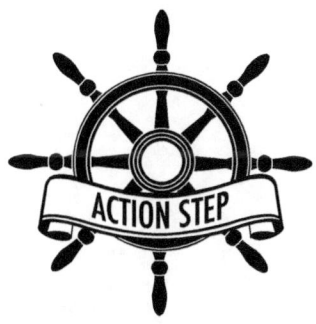

Look at the list you made of passionate experiences. Pick one passion that led to a success in your life. List any obstacles you overcame on the road to that success. What steps did you take to move over that obstacle? How did your passion fuel that triumph? Listing steps you take in success in various areas of life expands your concept of what time and resources will be required for you to achieve success with similar goals.

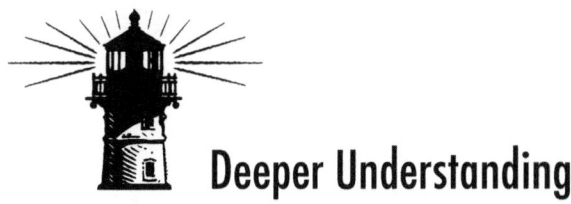

Deeper Understanding

My Voice Will Go With You—The Teaching Tales of Milton H. Erickson, Sydney Rosen, M. D., W. W. Norton and Co., New York, NY, 1982

DNA of Success Stories, Jack Zufelt (ed.), Z Publishing, Centennial Colorado, 2009.

How to Develop a Super-Power Memory, Harry Lorayne, Signet Books, New York, NY, 1974.

Think and Grow Rich, Napoleon Hill, The Ralston Society, Meriden CT, 1937.

Chapter 8
Time for the Life Preserver
(Save Yourself First)

*When something makes us sad,
we learn what's important to us.*
—Roy H. Williams

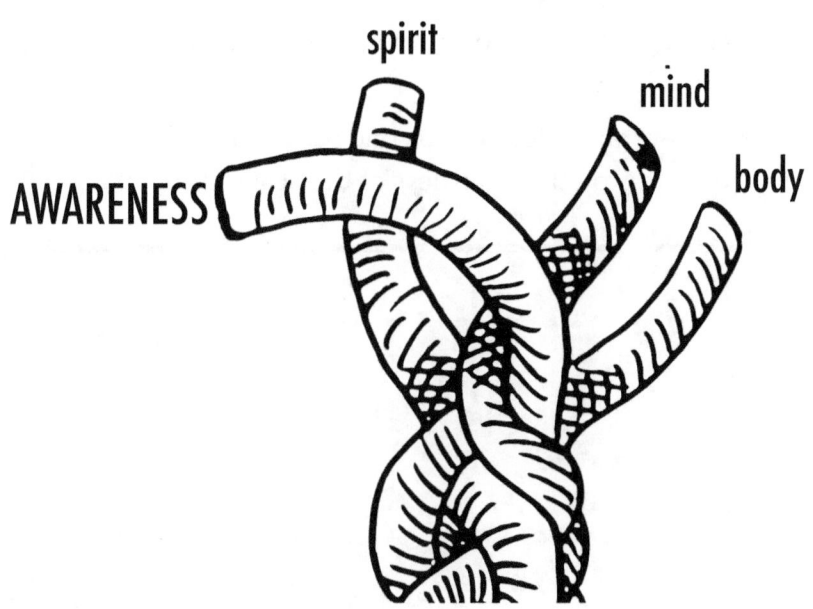

Lesson Summary

- Intuition, patience, and perseverance can be cultivated over time. These are especially useful when one is faced with an unexpected health challenge that has lasting effects.

- Intuition grows when you learn to ask the right questions and recognize when you can trust the answers you receive.

- Patience grows through expansion of the will, the ability to focus on one thought or object for an extended period.

- Perseverance develops as one passionately insists on self-growth, regardless of the obstacles.

Sal's Story

It is 1940, just after the Great Depression, and the United States is still trying to get back on track. Times are hard, especially in the rural areas, where many are still without electricity and doctors. A mother labors on the kitchen table to give birth in north Alabama. The mother's mother, a midwife, assists the only doctor in the county with the delivery. Both are stunned at this baby's appearance as she proceeds from the birth canal. The baby has no nose, bilateral clefts in the lip, and no roof of the mouth. How will little Sal survive? She cannot nurse because the nose and mouth form one large cavity, and babies must breath through the nose while feeding. The doctor sends the father to the drug store for a special nipple with a flap that seals the roof of the mouth. The father determines he will find treatment for Sal. Three days later the parents take the baby to a larger city to see Dr. Ledbetter, a surgeon. The baby returns home for a brief respite before surgeries that begin when she is three months old. Sal stays in the hospital the first two years of her life. Her parents stay with her most of the time while her two older siblings stay with their aunt. Sal leaves home a tiny baby and returns a beautiful little blond-headed toddler. Sal has 11 surgeries before she grows into a successful, self-confident 18 year old.

The roof of the mouth is difficult to repair while children are rapidly growing, so speech therapy starts when she is 11 years old. No speech pathology service is available in her rural town. Sal moves alone to a major university, hundreds of miles away from home, and stays in a university dormitory a full semester to improve her speech.

Sal becomes self-confident and self-sufficient as a child

and thus is totally comfortable with herself, her voice, and her appearance as she approaches adult life. As an adult, Sal takes classes at a business college and works for an optometrist for about 15 years. She marries a man who loves and appreciates her for who she is.

Despite a tough beginning, her brothers and sisters never hear her complain. As a child and to this day she is grateful for parents who sought the care she needed and provided an intense amount of love in a time when that level of care was uncommon in the rural South. Her great courage as a child molds her into a successful worker and loving wife, roles she enjoys very much.

Sacrificing Safety

Over time we develop skills that serve us when we encounter an unexpected health challenge that has lasting effects, like the birth of a child with a defect. Sal and her family applied liberal use of intuition, patience, and perseverance to their unexpected situation with remarkable results. Consider what the results can be without proper planning.

In a study of families with a child requiring a mechanical breathing machine to live, the family members struggled to lead a normal life. They felt as if they had been dealt an unfair lot in life and had no choice but to live it out as best they could. They had to give extra attention to the child with the ventilator, and the other children often were jealous. Family members felt isolated from society as a whole. Parents were overwhelmed with care delivery responsibilities they felt ill-equipped to handle. The families were shocked to find that society devalued the life of their child as someone whose life was not worth maintaining. While most individuals face the stress of death and the enrichments associated with miraculous survival on rare occasions, these families faced both every day. The cumulative distress took a toll on all family members.

Another study looked at the psychological and physical health of caregivers of children with cerebral palsy. In this study the psychological health of the caregiver was closely related to the presence and severity of child behavior problems. Daily caregiving demands affected the physical and psychological health of the caregivers. Self-perception, social support, and family function were also factors in caregiver health. Sal's family did not escape these factors. Instead, they used their common-sense intuition, which served them well as land stewards, and their faith to ensure that through patience and perseverance everyone in the family would be blessed.

Develop Your Intuition

Sal's family farms. They are tied to nature and their land. They understand the natural signs of life and its cycles and have a deep faith in their Creator. This type of lifestyle allows the right-brained intuitive nature of a person to flourish. Our technological advances insulate us from the natural cues of life and blunt the use of the right hemisphere. How do you reacquaint yourself with your gut instinct, your intuition?

The first step is to understand how this intellectual function likely works. Philosophers agree that on some level there are absolute truths that humanity in general recognizes. Consider this phrase, "We hold these truths to be self-evident." A part inside each of us resonates with absolute truth. If we can recognize when our physical body and mind agree with absolute truth, we can tap into our intuition at any time. Many different methods are used to measure the body's response to truth. There is the lie detector test, a variety of eye movement cues, and several forms of muscle-strength testing that can be performed.

One easy method is to start asking yourself questions that can be answered unambiguously and then listening to the yes or no answer that you receive first from yourself. For example, on a completely cloudless day, ask yourself, "Yes or no. Is the sky blue?" You will get an unambiguous yes by either listening to your inner voice or looking for some sign of muscle tension that you train yourself to recognize.

Next, ask yourself something obviously untrue like, "True or false. Is my mother George Washington?" Listen for the inner voice or recognize your negative muscle cue. Once you get used to hearing or recognizing some obviously positive and negative responses, you can begin to train yourself on simple intuition tasks that have no adverse outcome if your instinct is not completely accurate.

Action Interlude

Set an alarm to alert yourself after five minutes. Focus your mind on a candle flame, flower, or spot on the wall to the exclusion of all other thoughts. Repeat this exercise until five minutes becomes easy. Gradually increase the amount of time until you master a full hour. Then practice the same focus under increasingly complex conditions, such as a crowded mall or noisy restaurant.

You might explore traveling to a place you have never visited in town when you do not have an appointment deadline, using only the address and zip code and your instinct at each turn. Remember to listen to your first answer when you ask the unambiguous questions such as, "Right or left if I want to find the hobby shop?" The trouble arises when you start to allow your deductive reasoning faculty to intellectualize about the answer. That results in a left-brained, logical response. Strive to develop your right-brained responses with these exercises.

Patience and Perseverance

Some parents drop everything when an unexpected health challenge threatens a child. They leave work, family, and home to take care of the child. While this may cause short-term resentment in the siblings or spouse left behind, the example of patience and perseverance over time has a lasting effect on the other loved ones. It reinforces the idea that even the weakest member of the family deserves the best we have to offer. It subconsciously reinforces the idea of abundance because all family members learn that there is enough love, food, and support for all to enjoy.

You may see yourself and others as impatient. Patience and perseverance grow when faith in the outcome is fueled by passion. The intellectual faculty behind patience and perseverance is your will. The will is the ability to focus the mind on one idea or object for an extended period. When you become engrossed in any subject, time expands for you and allows you to enjoy the experience as if no time passes at all. Strengthen your will by meditation or prayer activities. Patience is the habit of watchful acceptance that what you expect will come to pass in due time. Perseverance is the habit of continuing to take the necessary action steps toward your goal even when circumstances do not look favorable.

The endurance of both patience and perseverance varies with the strength of your will. Be steadfast in will exercises and amazed at the grace you display as you wait for your health improvements to fully bloom.

Prayer Potential

The act of prayer has amazing healing properties and is often underused in formal health-care settings. One factor to consider about prayer is how it helps the person praying to learn to ask the right questions. Jesus made a big point of teaching his disciples an effective way to pray even though each man already was adept at prayer. One does not appeal to a Higher Power in the same way one asks a sibling to share a cookie. Instead, each question is respectfully worded with recognition of the action potential behind the request. In other words, one who learns to pray with the faith, reverence, and gratitude as if the request has already been granted infuses energy into the request. That energy resonates with like frequencies outside of the requestor and helps to attract the desired result. Ask audaciously and thank God with the delight of one who didn't deserve it and yet received it. You will live amazed at the blessings. Asking in any other manner demonstrates a lack of faith in God's limitless abilities. Never underestimate the power of the spoken word.

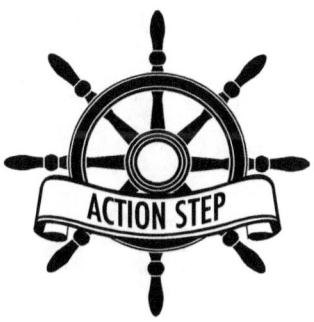

Walk barefoot outside on a natural surface: sand, grass, soil, or water. Stop, close your eyes, and attune your mind to sensory cues that help guide your intuition.

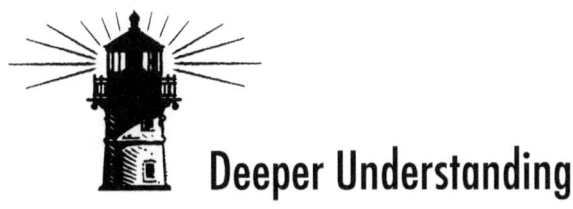

Deeper Understanding

"Daily living with distress and enrichment: the moral experience of families with ventilator-assisted children at home." by Carnevale et al. in *Pediatrics*, January 2006.

"The health and well-being of caregivers of children with cerebral palsy," by Raina, P et al. in *Pediatrics*, June 2005.

Gut Feelings: The Intelligence of the Unconscious, by Gerd Gigerenzer, Penguin Group, New York, NY, 2007.

Power Vs. Force, by David R. Hawkins, Hay House, Carlsbad, CA, 2002.

Chapter 9
Spiritual Mastery
(Live Up to Your Word)

*Think not of what you see but of what
it took to make what you see.*
—Benoit Mandelbrot

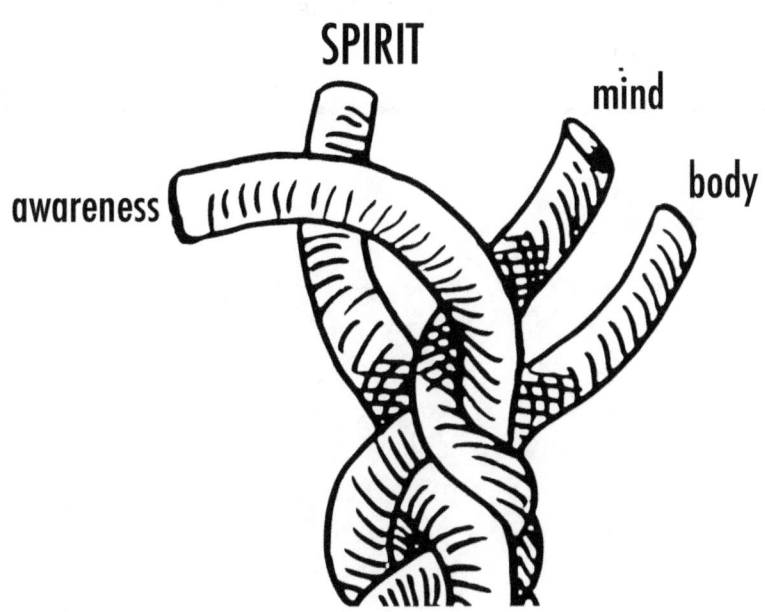

Lesson Summary

- Ordinary people sometimes have extraordinary, unexplainable experiences. This highlights that we are spiritual beings and that we have a body.

- Spiritual mastery involves total acknowledgment of our spiritual nature, from whence it arises and how it connects us with everything seen and unseen.

- As our faith expands beyond the bounds of what we are capable of as individuals, spiritual mastery solidifies.

Sonny's Story

Sonny begins to read when he is two and is encouraged to learn even though he is younger than his classmates in New Orleans. Times grow tough, and the family returns home to Alabama where educational standards are more about rules than individuals, and he is forced to conform. He is not allowed to attend school again until he is six years old. His ambidextrous tendencies are forcibly curbed, and he becomes a right-handed writer. He grows through reading, and reads whenever he can. Close friendships form with a few friends and relatives with whom he walks to school, works in the fields, and goes on boyhood adventures in the woods. He leaves his widowed mother at 14 and works as a riverboat hand.

When that proves to be less like Huckleberry Finn's story than he expects, he becomes a baker's apprentice in Chicago. He works hard, sleeps hard, and faithfully sends money home to support his family. By 16 he teaches himself enough algebra to finish electrician school successfully. He returns to Alabama only to find that the union will not admit him even as an apprentice because he is so young. At 17 he lies about his age and joins the United States Coast Guard. The structure of the military organization provides a social network where Sonny can thrive. He rapidly advances ranks. On a visit home to Alabama, he is touched by the message of a Christian preacher and is baptized in accordance with the Word of God. Reading takes on new depth, and Sonny begins to grow spiritually. He marries and continues to advance in the Coast Guard. His commanding officers recommend him for Officer Candidate School. He excels and advances as an officer.

His ship patrols the Gulf Coast in 1956 during Hurricane Flossy. Extensive damage mars the southern states of Mississippi and Louisiana. It is a rough passage of time on the water during the storm. He knows his wife is worried. When they arrive at the dock, the ship's captain will not allow any of the officers or crew to disembark. Sonny is furious. He knows what a relief it will be to the men serving and the wives at home to know that each other has survived. His anger is fierce. He picks up a phone and dials his home phone number. The phone rings; his wife answers. He says, "I am all right." She replies likewise, and they reaffirm their love. After he hangs up, he notices a queer fact. The phone is not wired to the wall. Somehow he has communicated on a nonphysical level during a highly charged moment. He and his wife tuck this information away and ponder it in private as the years pass.

Visited by Friends

Sonny retires after a full military career, in the city that inspired his self-sufficient childhood, New Orleans. He takes a sales job in the marine-repair industry. After some years, he and his best friend build their own repair and maintenance company that serves primarily the large number of cargo vessels and the companies along the docks of the port city. They enjoy their business and the comforts great success affords.

One night, as Sonny sleeps, he is visited by two of his childhood companions, both of whom have already passed on. If it is a dream, it is the most vivid of his life. They both urge him to "run, when the time comes, or you will wind up like us." He certainly remembers the dream in the morning and ponders it considerably.

A few days later just before dawn, Sonny is driving to their machine shop in New Orleans East. His car engine falters as he waits for the light to turn green. As he tries to start the engine, a car slowly approaches, and a young man armed with a handgun gets out. He is no stranger to Sonny's habits although Sonny doesn't know the man. Somehow he knows that Sonny is carrying the cash for the business and has engine trouble. After he takes everything of value he sees, he shoots Sonny in the side and closes the driver side door. His partner who is driving the getaway car says, "Shoot him again. He's not dead!" The assailant complies. The bullet penetrates the door window and strikes Sonny's head on the left side as he slumps to the right from the first wound. The bandits leave and Sonny faces his mortality.

The first shot has shattered his left arm bones, then penetrated the abdomen. With the second bullet to the head, he waits to die. Suddenly, he remembers his childhood friends. He is certain that this is the moment to which they referred. Sonny gets out of the car and begins to run. He is about a mile from the shop. He moves through dense weeds to the railroad track and runs, hoping his bloody tracks will not give him away. When he hears a car's engine approaching, he stretches flat on the tracks and holds his breath. When silence returns, he runs some more. Sonny approaches the night guard's post bloody and breathless. The guard fails to recognize him or believe him when he tells him his name. He thinks he is just an unfortunate drunk. Nevertheless, the guard calls an ambulance. Sonny breathes a prayer of thanksgiving that he survives this attack and prays for strength as he recovers. He is taken to Charity Hospital where instead of attending the party planned that day to honor his many hours of volunteer service, he lies on an emergency room gurney, low on the triage list for attention despite the head and abdomen injuries.

Spiritual Mastery Explained

In reading an earlier chapter, you remembered that you are more than just your body. You have a body. You really are a spiritual being. Your body is an instrument you use on earth. Coming to grips with your spiritual side causes feelings of both anticipation and anxiety. The spiritual nature of man can be a difficult concept. My father's story—he is Sonny—helps you to see life events that point to our spiritual self and to grow with that until you reach a point of spiritual mastery. Mastery is the ability to give yourself a command and follow through regardless of your circumstances. It is a reflection of your level of self-discipline. Spiritual mastery is one of the highest levels of self-actualization known to humankind.

Spirit is more than what animates our bodies. Spirit identifies us as children of God. Spirit is the perfect part of each of us, made in the image of God. Soul is the unique part of our spiritual self that identifies us as spiritual individuals. If we would focus on the spirit of those we encounter instead of their physical shortcomings, we would soon find a dramatic improvement in all of our relationships. Recognizing the perfect part inside of another human is the highest form of compliment. This act allows the individual's spiritual nature to be freely and fully expressed.

What is the role of spirit? Your spiritual side is the part of you that is involved with every connection you make, internally and externally. It allows your thoughts to communicate with your body. It allows you to have an intimate relationship with your husband or wife. It allows you to brush the thoughts and minds of all others inhabiting this universe. Your spirit sparks all growth and achievement. What gives your spirit all this power? Your spirit is created in the likeness of the Infinite Source. The more you align your spirit with this unlimited power, the more you will find you are naturally more susceptible to receiving the answers you seek. Sonny didn't need a working telephone after the hurricane. What he needed was to reconnect with his wife. Spirit provided a means for that connection. Neither Sonny nor Lee, my mother, is a metaphysical thinker, nor do they consider these events miraculous. They are simply Americans who appreciate the gifts they are given and who have faith that their needs will be provided through proper application of these gifts or blessings. They express their gratitude through faithful prayer. Providence works to their advantage since they are aligned with God's Word.

Sonny didn't need a visit from his dead friends. What he needed was to know how to survive an upcoming attempt on his life. Spirit provided that information. What is the key to developing this kind of spiritual potential?

Action Interlude

Recall an experience where you were able to inexplicably communicate with someone else without the aid of a telephone, fax machine, or the Internet. What emotion ignited that ability to communicate?

Faith is the Mystery

The real secret to unleashing your spiritual potential is the development of faith. Sonny's faith didn't germinate until he became an independently thinking young man. Faith develops only through understanding and study of ideas that are worthy of your deepest commitment. It is worth your while to study the lives of men and women who successfully operate from a strong faith-based position. Some of the most dramatic accounts of the power of faith as it works in a person's life are recorded in the Bible. While the first attempt to read some of these histories may result in confusion and misunderstanding, continued daily study will help you develop a familiarity with the thread of faithful individuals who are woven throughout the Word. Don't wait for a near-death experience like Sonny's to cause you to become serious about God's Word.

Practice Faith

The next step in the development of faith is to practice when it is easy to be faithful. If your life is full of blessings, thank the Provider every day. Appropriately expressed gratitude is a booster when one is in the process of deepening faith. Train your mind to be quiet during prayer, and be respectful in your approach. As you learn to quiet the mind at will, you discover that this skill carries over into any daily event. This leads to the next stage of development.

Next is to practice your faith when it is hard to believe. Tests of our faith make it stronger as we walk through life. The more of a habit you make of being a third-party observer with your quiet mind, the more likely you are to withstand harder trials of faith when they do occur. Just like Sonny, whose faith allowed him the freedom to think and live when he was shot, your faithful spirit will enjoy more options when trials arise.

Be Honest

The most important precursor to the development of faith is the ability to be honest with yourself. You can grow only in direct proportion to the amount of truth you are willing to handle about yourself. This is why the steepest curve in spiritual growth occurs once you are an independently functioning individual. Other folks can model faith for you, but only you can create solid faith within your spiritual self. Recognize that alignment and harmony with God increases your chances for survival during acute crises, such as the ones Sonny faced, and with long-term challenges to your physical existence, such as chronic disease. How is this possible? Faith creates hope, and hope allows room for improbable possibility. Look back once again at Sonny's story. How many individuals would have sunk into the car seat and relaxed into an easy death after being shot three times? His hope for survival was bolstered by his faith in the providence of God and by his understanding of how God's providence operates in the lives of human beings.

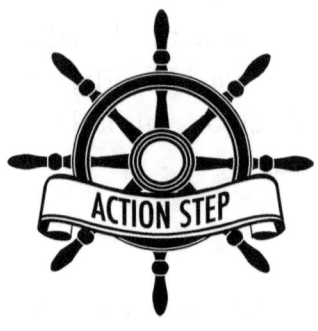

"What if?"

This one question is the most important question to ask yourself if you need to develop your faith. Use it as you read and study. For example, suppose you are reading the account of Jonah who was swallowed by the great fish and stayed in its belly for three days. Did Jonah know that a man could live inside a fish for three days? Probably not. Did Jonah have faith in the connection between himself and God? Absolutely so! Now ask yourself a what-if question in conjunction with what you read. Examples might be, "What if Jonah had no faith in God? Would the great fish have come?" "What if I had been Jonah?" Develop a habit of considering the what-if questions around different aspects of your life. Then let your imagination actually follow the path the what-if question creates.

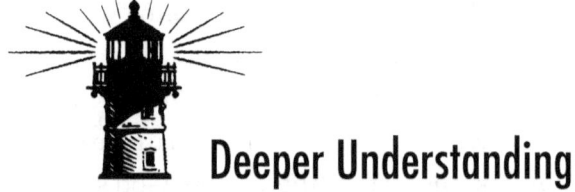

Deeper Understanding

Read or Listen to the Bible. F. LaGard Smith did a masterful job of arranging the text in chronological order and dividing it into 365 meaningful segments. *The Daily Bible*, Harvest House Publishers, Eugene, OR, 1999.

Healing Words, Larry Dossey, M. D., Harper Collins, New York, NY, 1993.

Flow: The Psychology of Optimal Experience, Mihaly Csikszentmihalyi, Harper and Row, New York, NY, 1990.

Chapter 10
Physical Mastery
(Fat Off Fast)

I am convinced that a light supper, a good night's sleep, and a fine morning, have sometimes made a hero of the same man, who, by an indigestion, a restless night, and rainy morning, would have proved a coward.
—Lord Chesterfield

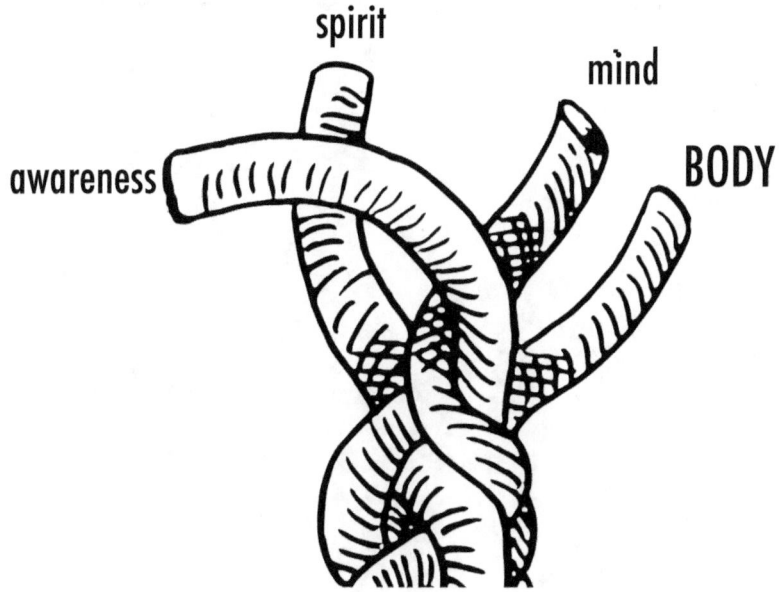

Lesson Summary

- Physical mastery begins with a new mental image that is reinforced by repetition.
- Work out in your imaginasium as much as you work out physically if you want to quickly and thoroughly master the physical skill.
- Consider other physical activities besides sports as worthy of mastery.

Amy's Story

Amy flashes blond hair and blue eyes. Beautiful from birth and as she grew up, Amy is reminded of how much she looks like her mother at different ages. After several soul-searching years in high school, she discovers her inner beauty is as great as her outer beauty.

She marries and starts her family. After three children, she discovers that the words "baby fat" have a whole new meaning. Instead of her babies' bodies, her body sports the soft, cushioning substance that represents the physical form of stored energy. For her parents' forty-fifth wedding anniversary, an album is planned. Amy is a scrapbooking expert. In putting together the scrapbook, she finds several pictures of herself in a bathing suit on the beach. She takes action and improves the look of those pictures so that they are in keeping with the image she wants for herself. She literally trims her thighs by cutting away the excess fat from the pictures.

At the anniversary party, her family admires the album. One of her sisters comments, "Amy, I don't remember you being quite so thin that summer." Amy readily admits, "Oh, I trimmed my thighs." Her sister pouts because her own thighs are accurately captured in the photograph.

Not long after this event, the excess energy that Amy stored on her body melts away easily. How did this work? What cemented Amy's perseverance to make this permanent release of weight successful? After all, Amy is like so many women; she gives more time to her family than she does to herself. She is over 35, very busy providing for her family, and has little time for physical exercise. Out of all of her family, she is the most successful at maintaining an ideal body weight and resisting the desire to store excess energy. The key lies in the act of physically trimming her thighs from the photograph.

Create a New Image

To understand why Amy's physical action helps to trigger a larger success that she may or may not have been conscious of, we must explore the question, "What really controls your physical body?" Recall that your body is an instrument to be used for the physical expression of your spiritual self. Your mind controls your physical body. We consciously allow thoughts, feelings, and actions to influence our subconscious mind. The subconscious mind is the storehouse of feelings. When we reinforce feelings, they form habits. When habits are reinforced, they form paradigms. Our paradigms about ourselves are some of the strongest we carry. Our physical body is a reflection of all of our thoughts, feelings, and actions. It is the physical manifestation of your attitude.

Notice how quickly a child's body changes from year to year. The mind of a child has many changeable ideas and many less-fixed thoughts than adults have. As thoughts become fixed, the body becomes less flexible. Over time certain body features become more prominent. For example, a person who makes a habit of being critical or angry carries furrow lines between the brows. A person who makes a habit of laughing develops crow's-feet at the corners of the eyes. The person with a poor self-image usually shakes hands with a hesitancy that reflects it. You leave the encounter feeling as if you have just grasped a cold, dead fish rather than a useful tool of a warm, vibrant person. A person who honors her body as an important representation of who she is usually has a fit body close to ideal weight with healthy-appearing skin and signs that the body is active. When you grasp the idea that one's body is a representation of the inner image that one carries in the subconscious mind, you think of many more examples of how a person's thoughts are reflected physically.

When Amy was scrapbooking, she had an opportunity to review pictures from all stages of her life. She revisited herself as a healthy baby. She enjoyed herself as a healthy teenager and remembered the emotional difficulties of her teen years. She saw herself as a beautiful bride. She saw herself as a loving mother. When she came to the pictures on the beach, she was startled because her memory of the vacations did not match what the pictures had captured about her body. While the memory was fresh in her mind, she took a physical action to make a change and trimmed the excess fat from her thighs on not one but several pictures. This act was so bold that it made an impression on her conscious mind that she freely admitted to her subconscious mind without any doubt that she was doing the right thing. The subconscious mind said, "Why, of course. Those thinner thighs are perfectly in keeping with the way I want to see myself." The subconscious mind felt perfectly in harmony with the new picture that Amy gave it to remember. Memories are stored associated with sensations, and one of the most powerful sensations we use to store memories is the mental picture.

Amy's subconscious mind filed away the new picture and the great feeling accompanying her improvement of her body in the picture. This was reinforced by Amy's renewed desire to achieve her ideal weight and release excess energy to the Universe. Her mind set up a new vibration, a healthier vibration. This higher frequency resonates with her body and with her environment. Her body had no choice but to follow through with actions that supported the new idea, reinforced by the image physically in the scrapbook, which she continued to work on for months. The idea was also reinforced by the strong emotions of pleasure from changing an unpleasant memory to a pleasant memory, by trimming her thighs in the scrapbook, and by her desire to achieve what she had lost by the storage of excess energy. This process guaranteed Amy success in her weight-loss goals.

Current Results Do Not Dictate Your Potential

Most people acknowledge their current physical circumstances and fix their subconscious mind on their present results. If I am currently carrying 50 pounds of excess weight on my body, and I see this on my body every morning in the mirror as I dress and when I get out of the shower, this is an opportunity for that physical image to be reinforced in my subconscious mind. If I am not mentally and physically taking steps to implant a new, healthier image in my subconscious mind, the subconscious mind is unlikely to create the vibration necessary to sustain my desire to release the excess energy.

Since most people don't recognize this factor, they live in a world of excuses. What is the truth about excuses? Excuses are messages we tell when we choose not to act. Excuses also serve as a way to tether us to one point in time or to a certain behavior. It is an omission of our responsibility for our circumstances in our lives. The only thing worse than a good excuse is a great excuse. When we remain fixed or stuck for a certain period, we begin to believe that we do not have what it takes to move forward. Sometimes we need a series of mental exercises to jump-start the process of movement before our physical body will follow.

Action Interlude

Name one new physical habit you will acquire: eating healthfully, increased exercise, more frequent and more fulfilling intimate relations, learning a new skill such as playing pool or painting; choose any physical activity.

On a piece of paper, list ten reasons why you have not already pursued a new habit. Spend a few minutes prioritizing your excuses because that's what they are: excuses. If you have difficulty prioritizing the excuses, look for the one that you think keeps you fixed and unmoving the most. After you identify it, ask yourself, "If this were not a factor, what would be the next thing that would stop me from moving forward?" When you have gone through your list, ask yourself if there is any other factor that keeps you from moving forward. The goal is to identify any excuses that are standing in your way.

Now go back and take another sheet of paper, and think about something you are pursuing or have relentlessly pursued in the past. Perhaps it is always making sure your children are in bed at a certain time or always making sure you worship God in a faithful assembly or always making sure that you have time for that date with your husband or wife. Now look at your list of excuses and identify what it is you do so that these excuses do not keep you from following through on the thing you desire most. These are the same skills you will employ as you develop your new habit.

At the end of this exercise, you will have a list of prioritized mechanisms that you employ to keep yourself from getting stuck. This is a very valuable list no matter what new endeavor you pursue until you develop enough desire, faith, and persistence to carry on without employing strategies. In other words, these are the skills that you help yourself with until your new desire becomes a fixed habit.

Visit the Imaginasium

Any chapter on physical mastery would be incomplete without a visit to the imaginasium. Until you have mastered the basic skill set necessary to develop your new habit, you will need to use strategies like the action interlude to assist you. If you want to make the most rapid progress in forming the new habit, act out success in the new endeavor in your imaginasium. Take yourself for a visit, and watch yourself as an expert in the physical endeavor you desire. Mental imagery is strongly employed by masters in many sports. Any great athlete not only sees himself making great shots every day but also actually visualizes the next shot successfully before taking each shot. People who master their physical body develop their creative imagination to a level where it serves them continually and unconsciously. They have a habit of seeing their success physically all the time.

When I was in medical school, Jane Fonda reinvented herself from being a shallow screen star known for her voluptuous curves into a true women's advocate through fitness videos. One of her favorite phrases was "Do you feel the burn?" When you work out in your imaginasium, the intensity of your imaginative visualization should be such that you feel the burn as you mentally sculpt your body. When you can feel the burn mentally, you'll find that the burn has more of an effect on your physical body.

Sports Aren't the Only Physical Activity

People equate physical mastery with proficiency in a sport or in exercise. While these are two areas where it is greatly beneficial to attain physical mastery, expand your perception and begin to view any physical activity as an area for potential mastery. Activities such as cooking, entertaining, tai chi, yoga, walking, corresponding, polishing, carving, and playing chess all are worthy of your consideration. Avoid being the "jack of all trades and master of none." Select one or two areas and devote the time, persistence, and will necessary to master those activities. Like Amy, trim your thighs and teach your subconscious mind a new idea.

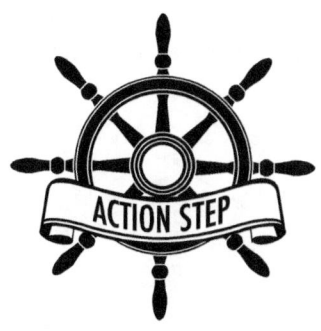

Consider an area with relation to your physical body where you would like to see improvement. Consider how many times a day, a week, a month, or a year you actually think about yourself in a very vivid way as already successful in that field. The frequency that you determine will help you understand how long it will take to become successful in that area. If you are giving thought to yourself as a success in this area only once a year, this idea is of such low priority in your subconscious mind—a mind that processes thousands of thoughts, millions of thoughts in a matter of minutes—that it will never manifest in your physical body within the course of your lifetime. It must come to the forefront of your subconscious mind. Make a commitment to think about yourself and visualize yourself as already successful in this physical endeavor at least once a day. When you have mastered the once-a-day habit, switch it to once every eight hours. When you have mastered the once-every-eight-hours habit, switch it to once every four hours. When you have mastered the once-every-four-hours habit, change it to once an hour. When you have mastered the once-an-hour habit, change it to once every 30 minutes.

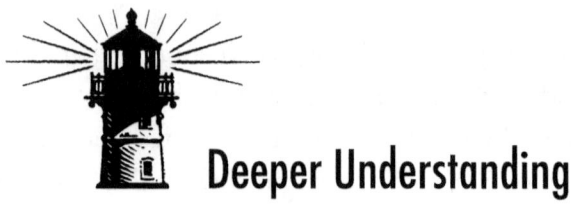

Deeper Understanding

Harvey Penick's Little Red Book: Lessons and Teachings from a Lifetime of Golf, by Harvey Penick, Simon and Schuster, New York, NY, 1992.

Search the web for renowned golf mentor Mike O'Leary. Pay attention to how he makes great golf an attainable habit for any person with motivation using his simplified swing and perfect power golf techniques.

Chapter 11
The Scientific Establishment Versus You (Examine Your Doctor)

The doctor of the future will give no medicine, but will interest her or his patients in the care of the human frame, in a proper diet, and in the cause and prevention of disease.
—Thomas A. Edison

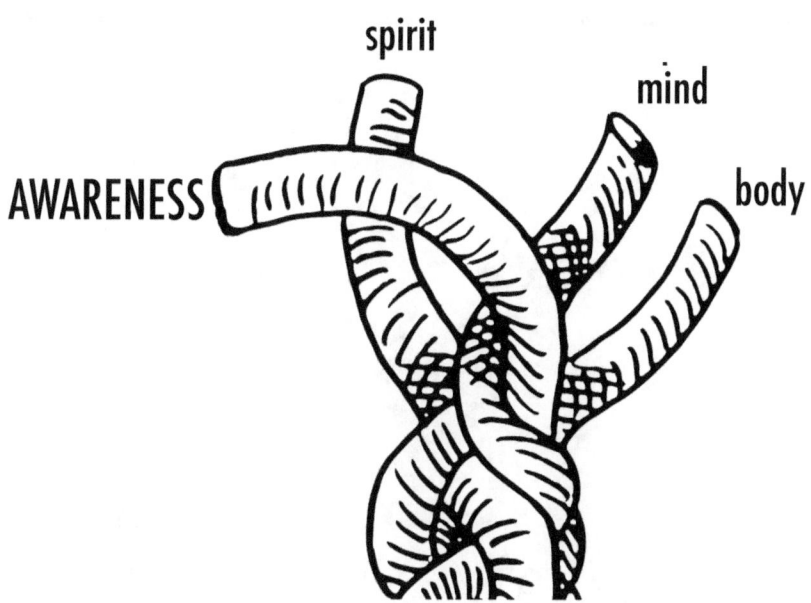

Lesson Summary

- The medical establishment is a very powerful voice we receive information from through our sensory factors.

- It is our responsibility to choose to accept, reject, or neglect their ideas regarding our health with our conscious mind to protect our own ideas of health in our subconscious mind.

Lee's Story

It is my second year of medical school, and the focus changes from learning the new language of medicine to actually learning about anatomy, physiology, and disease of the human body. We spend a great deal of time learning about the brain and how it functions. At one point in the study of neurophysiology, we cover Broca's speech area, an area of the brain thought to be critical for communication integration. Our instructor informs us that if an individual suffers a stroke and it affects Broca's speech area, the individual will never be able to speak again.

My mother is a career speech pathologist. She had taught stroke victims how to regain their voice for 25 years through the country's first home-health agency in New Orleans and has just returned to the public school system to teach children with speech impediments how to overcome these obstacles. That night, home from my classes and finished with my studying, I call her. I am excited because I'd learned about the part of the brain that she liked to reprogram. I tell her what I learned about Broca's speech area and its function, and I tell her what the instructor said, that if someone has a stroke in that region they would never learn to speak again. I will never forget what happens next. My mother begins to laugh in a way that reveals she has encountered this joke before. Finally, she says, "Now, Lori, you know that is not true."

She reminds me of how many patients she has treated over the years who had strokes that wiped out Broca's speech area and who subsequently, through faith and therapy, regained their speech. She reminds me of how plastic the brain is and how many portions of the brain are underused but can be reprogrammed through practiced, spaced repetition. The most important lesson, although not directly uttered, is that not everything I am learning in medical school is true. Until that point I have felt as if the information I have learned in medical school is the pinnacle of my education and absolutely true. Her simple statement reminds me that all knowledge is fallible and that wisdom supersedes knowledge in every instance.

The Scientific Establishment Resists Change

From a medical perspective, we are living in an exciting time, meanwhile, the world seems smaller because of mass media and cyberspace communication. Individuals are now able to understand both knowledge and wisdom from different cultures in a more integrated fashion than ever before. Yet the prevailing ideas, specifically in medicine and generally in science, are founded upon the Scientific Theory. This theory is based on independent observation of cause and effect through experimentation. One plans an experiment, carries out the experiment, makes observations recording factors that might have skewed the results of the experiment, and interprets the results based on the effect of the current experiment in light of history from related experiments. This forms the basis of most of the knowledge we call science.

As our global boundaries shrink, we are now able to appreciate wisdom-based practices that rely more on the intuition of the patient and the practitioner as worthy of our merit. Allopathic medicine, the common form of medical education employed in the United States, teaches doctors in training how to ameliorate the symptoms of a patient's disease. In other words, we fix flats. We do not build better tires that resist flats. In other cultures the focus is on staying well. They manufacture puncture-resisting tires. Thankfully, we are on the cusp of blending multiple disciplines so that patients can truly take responsibility for their own health and benefit from the wisdom of both practices that have been in existence for many years.

Even though the potential for wellness is vast and exciting, the process of changing mass thought in any area is glacially slow. The scientific establishment embraces change more slowly than most other disciplines. Take, for example, the story of Ignaz Semmelweis, the forward-thinking father of modern antiseptic technique. In 1847 this astute obstetrician noticed that one in ten women who delivered babies with the help of doctors and medical students who were performing autopsies died. When he forced the medical practitioners to wash their hands between the autopsies and the deliveries, this decreased to one in one hundred. He theorized that there were organisms that we could not see that were transmitted from the bodies of the dead to the bodies of the living on unwashed hands. When he reported his results to his colleagues in Vienna, he was dismissed from the hospital, ostracized by the medical community, and forced to move to Budapest. Even his wife believed he was insane. He was committed to an asylum, where he died. Only after his death was his theory proven, largely by the theoretical experiments of Louis Pasteur, and Semmelweis was vindicated.

The moral of the Semmelweis story is there is a high price to pay for thinking differently than the medical or scientific establishment. Many doctors and scientists have lost everything that they've gained professionally by embracing a new theory that they absolutely knew was true but that others could not see yet because of their own limited perceptions. Following are the names of just a few of the scientists who have suffered this fate.

- Galileo Galilei
- Albert Einstein
- Linus Pauling
- Abram Hoffer
- Robert Atkins

The Current State of the Scientific Mindset

More important to you, the potential patient, is the following question: What is the *current state* of the scientific mindset in the United States? (Emphasis placed on "current state" because there are pockets of individuals, professionals, manufacturers, insurers, and communities that are already transitioning into a more responsible model.) One needs only to follow the flow of the health-care dollar to answer that question. The independent American fed, a steady diet from food and drug manufacturers, insurance companies, and our well-meaning government, surrenders her health-care freedom and becomes enslaved to the dogmas of the system.

For example, the average American will accept only therapeutic regimens funded by insurance. If you wish to deny this fact, just look at the myriad of information regarding the benefits of large amounts of dietary fiber and the actual number of individuals who incorporate adequate fiber into their diet. We will spend billions on candy for Valentine's Day and yet love ourselves so poorly that we will not take fiber unless it is prescribed and our insurance pays the bill.

Insurance improves both quality of life and longevity, but it must be tempered with wisdom to take conscious action to improve our own health.

The prescription drug lobby is so strong and has influenced so many people and organizations that we see passage of startling legislation to limit the public's access to nutritional substances that have proven health benefits but that compete with expensive prescription drugs. We even focus our charity dollars on organizations that focus on disease treatment rather than prevention. Just look at the mission statements and funding histories of national, health-related, nonprofit organizations that come to call, and you will notice a telling lack of funding for prevention research.

Declare Your Health Independence

We as individuals must take full responsibility for allowing this to happen. It is only when individuals take responsibility for their own health and decide to make their own health-care decisions that there is pressure on the establishment to reconsider its omissions.

How do you recognize when your health-care system is working for you or against you? Start with your own perception of health. When do you choose to see a health-care professional? Is it only when you are sick, or is it while you are feeling healthy and you desire to know the best way to maintain optimal health? The answer to this question alone will reveal much about how you have been influenced by the current state of the scientific mindset. Are you open to training and education that inspires you to be responsible for the different aspects of your health? Let's say you have diabetes mellitus. Your doctor may prescribe insulin to control or to supplement what your pancreas can produce.

Your doctor may also ask you to follow up with a dietician for instructions on the best method of using food as your primary prescription for maintaining a healthy blood-glucose level.

Do you readily follow the dietician's advice? Are you savvy enough to recognize if the dietician is unduly influenced by governmental and scientific establishment guidelines for nutrition, or if the nutritionist is aware of recent research that supports a lower glycemic index diet with increased fiber and protein for diabetics? Do you do your homework before you visit a health-care practitioner? Are you aware of what your symptoms could mean and what the possibilities are so you can ask intelligent questions? Do you think of the possible answers the doctor might give you and what questions you might have should the need for further testing, surgery, or a referral be necessary? Once you have done your part to take responsibility for your own health, then is the time to assess the health-care delivery system in which you participate.

A good place to start is with your insurance. Insurance plans that support health over illness encourage individuals to live healthy lifestyles. Programs that allow individuals the freedom to choose if their health-care dollars are spent on nutritional supplementation, wellness programs, and effective screening tests are much more likely to produce wellness-centered results than are their counterparts that simply provide coverage for treatment of chronic illness and medical conditions requiring immediate surgery. A good alternative is a self-insured medical savings account that provides the same flexibility and some tax benefits for the self-employed. If you are insured by a government agency, you will need to be conscientious about providing documentation necessary to receive reimbursement if your care is not considered mainstream. If you are uninsured, you will need to develop a cooperative strategy to assure that you and your family listen carefully to your bodies for signs of dis-ease and avoid the habits that commonly degrade health in our culture: sedentary lifestyle, poor nutrition, and lack of meaningful activity.

The Two-Way Checkup

Next, consider your primary care provider. This may be a naturopath, a medical doctor, a nurse practitioner, or other qualified professional. Be aware of that person's training bias. If she was trained in an allopathic environment, the main idea of treating disease and ameliorating symptoms will permeate her professional thoughts. Usually this tendency is given away by the questions asked, such as, "Hello, Mrs. Sanchez, why don't you tell me what's bothering you today?" A person who has a more open mind about health and wellness will tend to lead with a question such as, "Hello, Mr. Wang, what brings you here today? What aspect of your wellness may I assist you with today?" If you are unsure, look for signs or directly ask what training your provider has received since obtaining her degree to learn about complementary therapies. If your primary provider gives you a stunned look and stammers for a response, be forgiving. It will take a while before every good doctor on the planet adjusts to the fact that their patients are now willing to take responsibility for their own health.

After every check-up of your own, make sure you give your doctor his or her own check-up. Almost every health-care practitioner, no matter what discipline, has customer comment cards available for feedback. Use these to communicate the ways your provider and staff can best meet your wellness needs. This is the way to reclaim your health independence.

Shield Yourself from a Fixed Medical Mindset

If you suffer from a condition that requires you to be in constant exposure to a fixed medical mindset, consider protective measures so that those pervasive ideas are less likely to seep in to your subconscious mind. As soon as possible, begin using your imagination to see yourself with the outcome you desire when you pass through the hospital, clinic, or office. Envision yourself as just a short-term visitor, never as an in-patient. Once you begin working with this picture of yourself, assign a positive word or phrase to the scene you envision so that whenever you hear that word, this scene permeates your conscious mind.

For example, assume you are a cancer patient visiting your oncologist's office for an afternoon of chemotherapy. Your imaginary visit might include a picture of pure golden

Action Interlude
Your Doctor's Check-up

Ask if there is a standardized form or web tool your doctor's office uses for feedback. If so, use it after every visit. If not, pick up a form from your favorite restaurant and use it as a template to create your own form to assess the visit. If you are uncomfortable submitting the information to the practice, make a vistit to your imaginasium where you imagine discussing the results with your provider.

energy infusing through your body while the intravenous fluids run. You might see the staff as spa personnel seeing to your body's every need. You might meditate and feel warmth rising from the easy chair in which you sit as you become grounded with the goodness of the earth. You might assign the word "renewal" to this vision, and you might begin speaking in those terms to the staff: "I am here to begin my renewal for this week." Most important, explore the value of laughter with regard to your health. Laughter is such a powerful tool and totally underutilized—especially inside health-care environments where individuals make a habit of taking themselves too seriously.

Take Healthy Action

Make a conscious choice to replace every thought, phrase, or experience that is counter to your desire and goal for health with a positive affirmation or vision or memory that supports the good you desire. Once you begin to protect your mind and reclaim your health independence, you will become aware of additional opportunities to support your independent wellness plan and let the scientific establishment support itself.

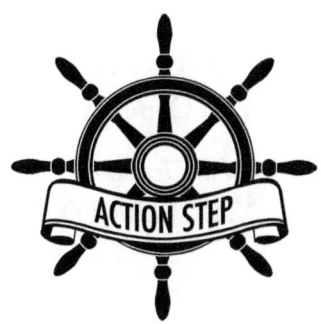

Visualize your ideal visit to your doctor or other health-care practitioner in the imaginasium. Build in sufficient detail to be able to experience the smells, sounds, and sights.

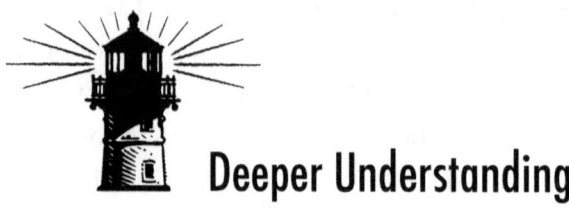

Deeper Understanding

Explore the reasons why any of these men chose to expand their view of science and medicine past the bounds of what they were taught.

Are there practitioners in your community who stretch the bounds of the medical establishment?

How are they viewed?

Galileo Galilei

Albert Einstein

Linus Pauling

Abram Hoffer

Robert Atkins

Why Our Health Matters, by Andrew Weil, Penguin Group, New York, NY, 2009.

Anatomy of an Illness as Perceived by the Patient, by Norman Cousins, W. W. Norton and Company, New York, NY, 1979.

House Calls, How We Can All Heal the World One Visit at a Time, by Patch Adams, M.D., Robert D. Reed Publishers, San Francisco, CA, 1998.

Chapter 12
The Gift of Appreciation
(Bottomless Gratitude)

La reconnaissance est la memoire du coeur.
—*Jean Baptiste Massieu*

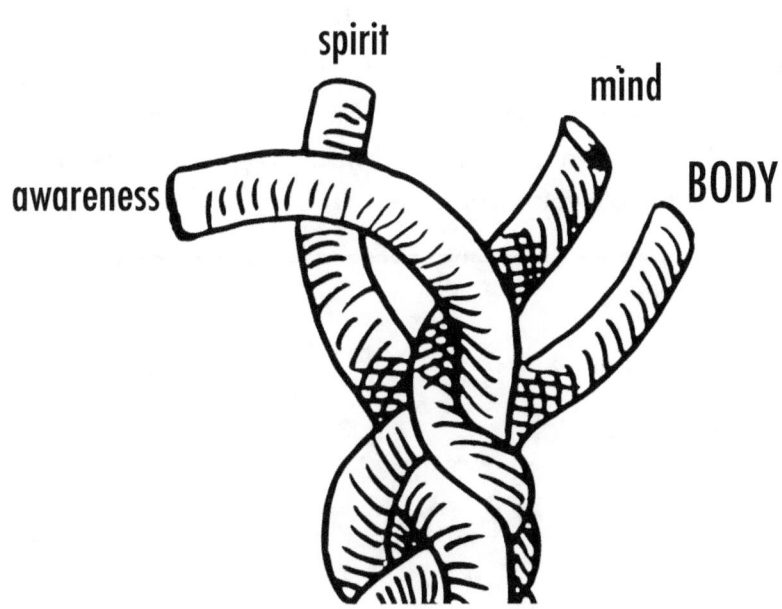

Lesson Summary

- Laughter is the result of not taking the importance of one's thoughts and actions too seriously.
- Gratefulness is the habit of expressing gratitude, thanksgiving, or appreciation, or causing gratitude or a welcome, pleasing feeling.
- Gracefulness is the habit of having grace or beauty of form, composition, movement, or expression.
- These characteristics have spiritual, mental, and physical components that are cultivated over time.
- Every human being has an innate desire to make a difference in the world. Are you recognizing this in the people you meet?

Lori's Story

After five years of marriage, my husband and I decide it is time to start our family. The baby is due in March. Early pregnancy is a glorious experience that enlivens the senses of smell and taste. I enjoy a weekend in August when I meet my best friend and my mother in New Orleans. We spend the whole weekend visiting all of my favorite restaurants. I savor the intense flavors of all my favorite foods in a way only possible during pregnancy and am grateful to enjoy this pleasure.

In November I travel to Louisville, Kentucky, to prove my knowledge is sufficient for a certificate of added qualification in pediatric radiology from the American Board of Radiology. Shortly after returning to Cincinnati from this stressful examination, I feel more contractions than usual. My doctor times the contractions and starts me on a course of daily terbutaline until my pregnancy reaches 34 weeks.

Gradually, as the weeks pass, I learn to be more aware of my body's response to stress. I tuned that information out until the pregnancy brought it to my conscious mind with great intensity. I see my obstetrician every two weeks, and early in January he decides I am far enough along to take me off of the terbutaline therapy. Four days later, I am in the hospital with premature rupture of my membranes. The baby is six weeks early.

Within 24 hours the baby develops signs of distress, and an emergency caesarian section is performed. Since I ate a piece of pumpkin pie and drank a glass of buttermilk, I will not be asleep for the surgery. Instead I receive an epidural and have the unsettling experience of knowing too much of the surgical jargon that the on-call obstetrician and his trusty resident sidekick discuss as they carve.

I am naked, open, and cold beyond belief. With the intravenous line in one arm and the other arm away from my body as well, I am in a crucifix position. My upper torso is shielded from the sterile field so that neither my husband nor I witness the actual surgery, only the conversation and the sensation. My right hand, on the arm without the intravenous line, finds the only warm thing in my current realm of existence, and I cup my hand firmly around it taking great comfort from this small blessing. As the surgery concludes, the baby boy is safely delivered, and I am closed. Moments later the warm structure where I am resting my right hand moves. To my horror, I realize that my hand had grasped the backside of the chief resident for the duration of the surgery!

Perhaps the natural endorphins released during bodily stress made me say what I did. Perhaps it was the sheer frank gratitude I honestly felt for the warmth he unknowingly provided. As I moved to the gurney to be taken from the surgical suite, I said, "Dr. M., I want to apologize for having my hand on your backside during my surgery. I didn't realize it was you until now. I want to thank you because it was the only warm thing in this room, and it really comforted me." There was dead silence for about 30 seconds. Then we all broke out laughing. Gratitude is a beautiful thing, even in the most embarrassing situations.

The Beauty of Gratitude

How often have you been comforted by the actions of another individual who had no idea that he was comforting you? It happens to each of us, yet we rarely take the time to thank the comforter. Results of more than 300 studies on the health effects of altruism, with results varying from increased mental health to increased longevity, have been published. Some of the studies show health benefits for the person who is performing the act of kindness. Observers of the act of kindness also receive benefit. What is more, there are health benefits for the performer of the act in simply remembering the act of kindness.

Of particular interest is the 2003 research of Dulin and Hill, of Massey University in New Zealand, whose work demonstrates that elderly people who volunteer have increased longevity over those who don't. The factors thought to contribute to increased longevity were the sense of community one feels by giving, the lack of isolation, and the physiologic effects of giving on stress reduction and the stress mechanism. Smiling and laughter have also demonstrated remarkable effects on one's mood and physiology.

If you have not already established habits of laughing, sharing, and gratitude, how do you start? As with all new habits, the first step is to assess your current level of awareness and your current activity in this regard. You must grow to recognize opportunities where appreciation is appropriate. In general, people far underestimate the value of giving thanks and after age 40, laughter decreases.

As you increase your awareness of the art of thanksgiving, look for examples of people who have already mastered this skill. One client with whom I recently worked shares words of gratitude from such a deep place that they move large numbers to tears. She did not develop this skill haphazardly. She is grateful every day and multiple times a day on many levels.

> **Action Interlude**
>
> Identify someone within your community who is really great at laughter, gratitude and grace. Write down three gratitude expressions they use. Record three ways they are graceful and three ways they employ humor.

Three Levels of Thanksgiving

Regarding physical manifestations of thanksgiving, look at opportunities around you every day to make small gestures of appreciation or to show respect. This could be as simple as opening a door for someone or helping someone with a package. If you recall all of the admonitions given to Boy Scouts of examples of being helpful, you have a good idea of the small tasks that can make big differences over time. You will find as you develop a habit of physical gratitude, that you will find larger and larger ways to express this side of yourself. My friend Marcie Henna put it this way: "Giving leaves your hand open to receive."

Remember that giving thanks happens on three levels. There is the spiritual act of giving thanks, where we communicate with God through prayer. There is the intellectual act of giving thanks, where we say the words "thank you" and express our gratitude through communication for something that someone has done for us. There is the physical expression of gratitude by reciprocal action or by physically involving ourselves in an activity that expresses gratitude. A new habit of gratitude needs to be established on all three levels.

In the first letter he wrote to the Thessalonians, Paul the apostle encouraged us to "pray without ceasing." Becoming more mindful of our blessings helps us grow on the spiritual level. Develop a daily habit of prayer, and don't miss an opportunity to encourage the two-way communication between you and Infinite Intelligence. As we communicate gratitude to God, we become more open channels to receive His blessings through providence.

On the intellectual level, consider the advice of Earl Nightingale, who in his landmark program, Lead the Field, encourages the listener to "treat every individual as if they are the most important person in the world."

Perhaps you have met the president of the United States or have been in the presence of the queen of England. At the end of such an encounter, the natural response is to thank these people for the time they have granted you. Begin treating every human being with that same courtesy and respect every time you encounter someone. Try this for just one day. Be mindful of the importance of everyone you meet and of everyone's great desire to make a difference in the world. Share your gratitude for the difference each person makes in your life. This is one of the most gratifying feelings you can invoke in another person. It truly voices the love that you carry and share.

Grateful vs. Graceful

As you look for role models who are living a grateful life already, you will begin to notice that these same people live a graceful life. What is the difference between grateful and graceful? Grateful is either feeling or expressing gratitude, thanksgiving, or appreciation, or causing gratitude or a welcome, pleasing feeling. Graceful is having grace or beauty of form, composition, movement, or expression. Grace comes from the Latin *gratia* which is a pleasing quality, favor, goodwill, thanks, and is closely related to *gratis*, which means pleasing.

Recognize the Best in Others

Since the utmost need of individuals is to feel as though they make a difference and to be recognized for that, you will find as you cultivate your habit of gratitude that you will be perceived as more graceful. You will begin to recognize and appreciate when grace is extended toward you on the physical, intellectual, or spiritual level. This is one of the most meaningful areas of life in which you can grow. It is worth attention every day of your life and moves you closer to your life's purpose. During times of illness, it is easy to become self-centered and to focus on limitations. If a habit of grace is cultivated before the onset of illness, it changes the dynamic so strongly that sometimes illness is not even perceived as an obstacle.

Was I graceful in the delivery suite? Not by a long shot. But no one questioned my deep gratitude for every little thing done to support our family during this birth. Make sure you leave no questions behind as you become more grateful and gracious.

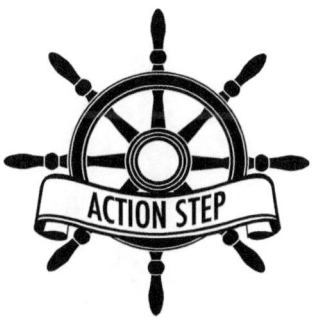

Begin a joy and gratitude journal. Faithfully write at least six things every day for which you laughed and/or are thankful. As you evaluate your list of six, identify whether gratitude happens on the spiritual, physical, or intellectual plane, and take the time to express it. List more than one plane if need be.

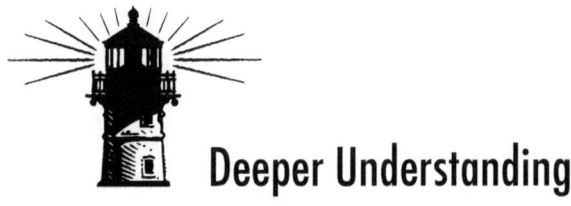
Deeper Understanding

"Relationships Between Altruistic Activity and Positive and Negative Affect Among Low-Income Older Adult Service Providers," by P. Dulin and R. D. Hill, in *Aging and Mental Health*, July, 2003.

"Humor and Laughter May Influence Health IV," by M. Bennett and C. Lengacher in *Humor and Immune Function, Evidence-Based Complimentary and Alternative Medicine*, 6(2):159-164, 2009.

I Thessalonians, by Paul the Apostle, in The Holy Bible, American Standard Edition, Nelson Publishing, Nashville, TN, 1901.

Lead the Field, by Earl Nightingale, Nightingale-Conant, Niles, IL, 1960.

Chapter 13
Let Go
(Kick Habits)

Happy the man who bears within him a divinity, an ideal of beauty and obeys it; an ideal of art, an ideal of science, an ideal of country, an ideal of the virtues of the Gospel. These are the living springs of great thoughts and great actions. Everything grows clear in the reflections from the Infinite.
—Louis Pasteur

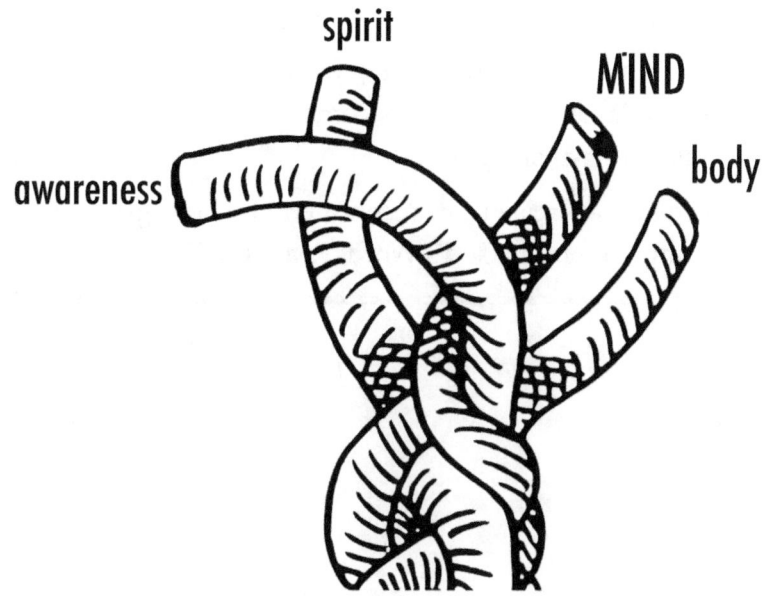

Lesson Summary

- Habits fulfill personality needs, and when a great number are filled by one activity, addiction occurs. To treat a negative addiction, use your will to identify the needs the addiction meets and to persist with new activities that fill that need until the addiction is gone.

- Holding on to both physical and nonphysical things that no longer serve us is addressed by consciously letting go.

- The yin and yang of holding on and letting go are always around us. They become more evident when it is our final struggle.

- The best exercise I can recommend for strengthening the will is God's Word. Read it daily.

Sam's Story

Sam is a forty-something successful anesthesiologist. He rises early and gets off from work early. His days are filled supervising a number of nurse anesthetists and the busy operating room suites of the hospital in which he primarily practices. In medical school, he was happy-go-lucky. He participated in a medical school, fraternity known for decadent parties, loose morals, and easy access to taboo excesses. He developed a habit of social drinking during college and continued that habit throughout medical school and his residency.

By the time he settles into his practice in a mid-sized metropolitan area, his life revolves around rising early, putting in his time at the hospital, getting off early, and spending the rest of his time having fun. It takes him a long time to decide to settle down. When he does marry, he marries a supportive nurse, Jenny, who provides some grounding for his free spirit. Nevertheless, as the workload continues to grow, Sam finds himself more and more dependent on his daily alcohol for stress relief. Eventually, he finds alcohol is not enough. With easy access to addictive substances used for anesthesia, he begins a dangerous habit of using the leftover bits of medicines that are supposed to be discarded. It is easy for him to support his habit. It is rare that the entire dose of a medication is used in surgery, and it is easy for him to pocket, rather than discard, the excess. One day when he is on call, an emergency surgery is scheduled just after he enjoys some of the medicines left behind.

One of his colleagues, the surgeon on the case, notices that Sam is impaired and turns his name in to the state medical review board. An investigation begins. Sam is tested for substances. He fails the urine test. Sam has a choice: lose his medical license, or enter a substance-abuse program designed to help individuals with these habits. Among the thousands of programs like this around the country, only a few have the reputation of successfully helping people set aside their addictions. It is a long, hard road. The people who succeed have an intense desire for change to be permanent. Luckily, Sam is enrolled in one of the best programs in the country.

The rigorous live-in program interrupts his practice, his family life, and his lifestyle. While he is enrolled, he is not allowed to leave the campus and not allowed external communication. When he moves to a halfway house, his wife files for divorce. She takes custody of their children and seeks a stable relationship. Sam learns that his practice partners now mistrust him. They are willing to give him another chance, albeit with close supervision.

Eventually he returns to his city and reintegrates into his medical practice. His local medical society and medical board provide weekly support. At one of the meetings with the psychologist, it's suggested that Sam attend a meeting of Alcoholics Anonymous. He does and is pleasantly surprised by the open, honest interchange with people who are not afraid to admit their weaknesses. He begins to make the weekly meetings a habit, and months pass to years. Every year that he remains sober and substance-free, he is rewarded with a small token, a chip that he carries in his pocket to remind him of his successes. Although he has lost many of the things that he worked hard to gain, this chip is the key that allowed him to leave his self-imposed prison. This has more meaning to him than any of the other things he lost.

Addiction Defined

Sam's story is a common picture of addiction among professionals in our country, but untreated addiction is far more prevalent. People become addicted to food, beverages, mind-altering substances, the Internet, video games, unhealthy relationships, and sports. Any activity in which a person engages for an undue amount of time and that takes away pleasure in other areas of life is an addiction. Addictive behavior is rooted on the foundation that the addiction fulfills some basic behavioral needs that are not being fulfilled by other aspects of a person's life. This is how people become addicted.

Any event outside of us that meets three or more of our six basic personality needs—certainty, variety, significance, love and connection, growth, and contribution—will meet our needs at a high level and can become an addiction.

Letting Go of Addiction

When you evaluate your habitual behaviors, it is important to assess which of these needs your habits address and to take note of those items that may be out of balance or an addictive behavior. Whenever you give up an addictive habit, such as smoking, it is important to identify which needs it has met and to replace those needs, which will no longer be met, to fill the void. Otherwise, you may reinitiate the same habit of smoking, or you may replace it with an even worse habit, such as overeating. True growth is found when you strike balances between your personality needs. Sometimes you must let go.

If you study individuals who are acclaimed for their level of spiritual awareness, you will notice a common trait.

Action Interlude

Write down any habits that do not serve you any more.

For each habit, identify which of these needs the habit meets: certainty, variety, significance, love and connection, growth, or contribution.

Map out a plan to meet these needs differently.

Try it for one day. If that works, try it for another day, then another and another. If that does not work, reassess your motives for the habit.

They are not trapped by material possessions. They could be very wealthy; however, they are the same person with or without their massive wealth. Many of them choose to give up nearly all of their physical possessions and to exist in a simplified state. This truly reflects their ability to honestly love and accept themselves for who they are without any dressing up by what they achieve or by what they accumulate.

Levels of Awareness

This is truly the larger scope of letting go. We move through different levels of awareness from the animalistic fight-or-flight level up to a level where we recognize we can make change and achieve the point where we can give ourselves a command and follow through, almost like Dorothy moving through the tornado in the Wizard of Oz. We can master transitions around material possessions and ideas by making space for the new and by letting go of the old. This is the ultimate form of letting go.

The Pinnacle of Awareness

So where is the pinnacle of awareness? Most people agree that the ultimate level of awareness is where you are able to view yourself irrespective of time or space, view your connectedness with God, and view your connectedness with all of the other humans who currently live, have lived, and will live. It is where you recognize your unique role in the world at the time you exist physically. You not only recognize it but also use your potential to its fullest. This is achieved only when you are able to view yourself honestly and when you are able to be completely transparent with other people.

People who attain this level of awareness usually spend a great deal of time in deep meditation or in communication with other people through unconventional means. Their level of faith and belief in the power of connectivity gives them abilities that most people would perceive as miraculous. If asked, most of these individuals will reveal that attainment of such mastery is indeed a simple process of self-discipline and it is not an easy path in life.

Harnessing the Will

Admit it. When you saw the chapter title, "Let Go," did the foggy breath of death whisper in your ear? Let's spend a moment examining possibilities with that form of letting go. In an earlier chapter you met Gene, one of two persons to whom this book is dedicated. Gene did wind up having a quadruple bypass back in 1979 at the time he quit smoking.

He exercised and watched his diet with the help of his wife. Five years later he had a triple bypass. Just a few years ago he underwent coronary artery stenting because the grafts had started to narrow again from plaque. In the spring, his wife, Edith, suffered a medical illness that required hospitalization. When she came home from the hospital, Gene took care of her needs. Three days later he began having chest pain and rushed to the emergency room. Even though he did all the right things, his time tunnel was about to close. While there, he suffered a massive heart attack. Using his will, he remained spiritually, mentally, and physically present until his children and his oldest granddaughter could come say farewell. They came from all around the country for his last waltz. He danced with dignity, bowed with grace, and there was no encore.

Gene and Edith were realists. They took all the necessary steps to prepare for the inevitable. With Edith's recent release from the hospital, the focus was on her. Nobody expected Gene to leave the stage at that point. Even though

Action Interlude

Have you taken steps necessary to prepare others for your passing?

Do you have a living will?

Do you have a list of assets and how to access them?

What about your user names and passwords?

Eternal life is something different from just maintaining a social networking page indefinitely. Is your soul secure?

we know that death is inevitable, we always think the other guy will go first. What is remarkable is the way Gene harnessed his will for the 24-plus hours it took for his family to reach him. Gene was a disciplined writer. He knew what the will was and how to use it effectively. He had no doubt that his spirit lived beyond the bounds of his physical body and that he could maintain his presence if his desire was strong enough to provide the energy his body lacked. He was able to relax and focus on this one task because he had no fear about his soul. He knew he was prepared to sleep until the time when he is called to arise anew.

Holding On vs. Letting Go

Holding on to both physical and nonphysical things is a constant tug in the opposite direction of letting go. The yin and yang are always around us and become most evident as one prepares to pass on into a purely spiritual existence.

If you are unsure about the preparation of your soul for what lies beyond, let me tell you about Carol's dream. She dreams it is Judgment Day and she is standing before the Mercy Seat where Jesus is reading from the Book of Life. God calls her forward. He asks, "Tell me, Carol, what have you been reading?"

She replies, "Oh, I just finished the latest Danielle Steele novel."

"Have you been reading anything else?"

Carol names a few more books and a few magazines.

Then God looks her in the eye. "Tell me, Carol, have you ever read My Book?"

The morning Carol told me this story we were walking around our neighborhood in Ohio getting some exercise.

With the last line, I felt chills along my arms and legs. I stopped.

"Have you read the Bible all the way through?"

"Close to it once, but, no, not really."

"Let's start today," we agree. Even today, I continue to read it before bed at night before I read anything else.

Hold On to These Healthy Ideas

Reading the Bible takes patience to wade through some of the books, and it takes humility when it steps on your toes. The rewards are unparalleled.

When your six mental muscles—imagination, intuition, perception, memory, will, and reason—become as conditioned as individuals existing in the higher planes of awareness, you will find that all of the exercises that seemed so hard when you started *Journal to Think and Grow Well* are really no different from daily physical exercises like squats and pushups. Physiques range widely, and all have a few highlights and perhaps a few flaws. The assets of our spiritual beings likewise range widely. Your goal is to spend the time needed honing the strengths for both your physical body, the tool through which you interact with your world, and your soul, the part of you that carries over past the brink.

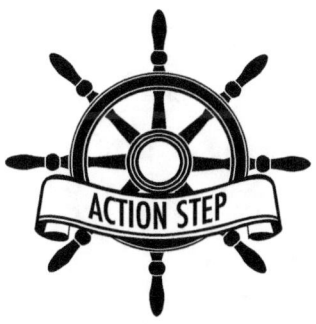

Think about Pasteur's quote. Have a conversation with someone you love about your desires when your life ends and his or her desires when life ends. Afterward, write a reflection of your feelings.

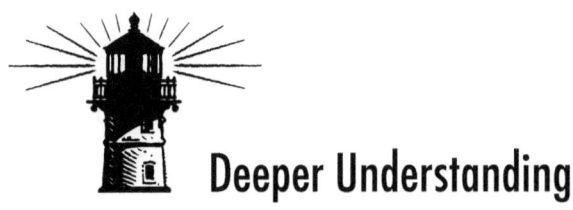

The Holy Bible, American Standard Edition, Nelson Publishing, Nashville, Tennessee 1901.

Human Scale Development: Conception, Application and Further Reflections, by Manfred Max–Neef, The Apex Press, New York, 1991.

"Six Human Needs," by Anthony Robbins, http://www.tonyrobbins.com/6HumanNeeds/
Listen to Tony simplify these needs and how we live them.

Alcoholics Anonymous, http://www.aa.org

Chapter 14
Cross the Finish Line
(Go Out in Style)

We don't die; we kill ourselves.
—*Sinclair Lewis*

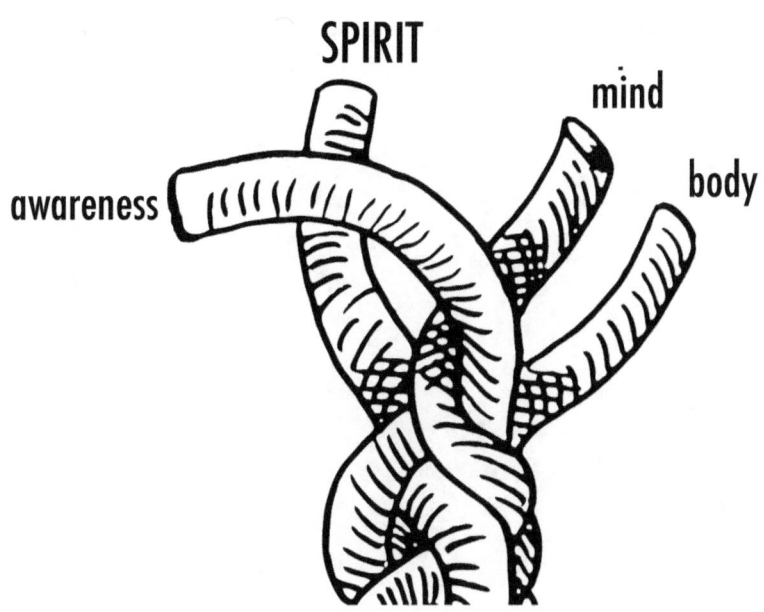

Lesson Summary

- Energy is depleted by law, our thoughts, circumstances and our reactions to others.

- Individuals become conduits for energy when they recognize it is abundant and ever-present.

- Increase your capacity to store energy by becoming passionately involved with one idea larger than your own existence.

Sonny's Story

A diagnostic radiology residency includes four years of mastery of image interpretation, radiation biology, nuclear medicine, and imaging physics. In my third year, I am reading skeletal X-rays with one of my favorite mentors, Mac Wilson. He is a brilliant physician with an astute eye and wry sense of humor. Every day spent with Mac is filled with learning about imaging and about life.

Midmorning, I get a phone call from my father, Sonny. This is about ten years after his shooting. He is in a state I had previously experienced only with patients. "Lori, the doctor says I have prostate cancer, and he wants me to make some decisions regarding treatment." Yet, when I try to get answers to more specific questions—like, "What Gleason stage is it?"—it is clear that he is in shock and unable to remember what the doctor said. I can almost smell the seared flesh from his new mental tattoo. Radical prostatectomy is the treatment of choice at the time. After further work-up proves no distant metastases, he chooses this treatment.

He undergoes the surgery in a training institution where medical students, residents, and fellows work side by side with seasoned physicians and surgeons. It is the time-honored tradition of medical education and is invaluable in the propagation of this healing art. Sometimes the teaching institution leads to a less personal encounter with the doctor from whom the patient seeks care. Certainly Sonny experiences this, bewildered by the number of people in white coats who present themselves to him and shocked to wake up after surgery with sutures and tubes in places he did not expect. Out of all those white coats, nobody shares that effect of surgery with him before his consent. He handles this indignity with grace, and a few days later learns that the cancer has spread to a few local lymph nodes. The recommendation from the oncologist and the urologist is radiation therapy.

His treatment plan is carried out over a period of weeks. Fatigue ensues, and he firmly believes this will lead to a cure. It does. But like everything else in life worth possessing, it comes with a price. In the prime of life, enjoying great personal and financial success with his own maintenance and repair business, he readily accepts lasting limitations from the surgery and radiation therapy.

He adjusts to these lifestyle changes with an uncommon grace and is soon back on the golf course playing and also conducting business with the charm and integrity that marks him as a good business partner.

Ten years later he is cured of his cancer and thus has the joy of growing older, transitioning to a more sedentary farming life. He enjoys his grandson and simple pleasures such as golf, fishing, and renewing the land. Twenty-three years after diagnosis, he is still cancer-free and maintains his momentum as a thinker, golfer, and farmer.

Health Setbacks

Why is it that some folks like Sonny never seem to have serious setbacks, whereas others seem overwhelmed by the smallest changes in their lifestyle? Sonny sees his share of setbacks, and he fully understands their cause-and-effect relationship. Mental, emotional, and spiritual setbacks occur for the same reason: energy depletion beyond our capacity to replenish.

Physical setbacks occur when we have depleted our

energy levels to a point that our body cannot recover normally. Three factors that contribute to physical energy depletion are inadequate deep sleep, poor nutrition, and decreases in mobility. While these factors are easy to identify, they also swirl into a catch-22.

If you are stricken with an illness that causes you chronic pain, it is unlikely you feel enough comfort to sleep as deeply as you need to for your body to produce the hormones it needs to maintain vitality. Pain also decreases your mobility and your ability to prepare good meals for yourself.

Energy Depletion

If you are already in the habit of eating a heavily processed diet rich in empty carbohydrates, you are at risk for metabolic syndrome, a condition where you do not effectively use your insulin for energy production. Less energy in, minus a constant energy flow out means gradual depletion over time. This results in feeling "just too tired" to move around as your body needs to maintain health. This leads to weight gain that is associated with sleep disorders. Are you beginning to see the catch-22 pattern?

Action Interlude

Watch the movie *Super Size Me* or read the book *Fast Food Nation: the Dark Side of the All-American Meal* (also a movie).

Explore the different types of energy in the universe.

Emotionally and Mentally Drained

Have you ever felt emotionally drained? Depletion of emotional energy is a familiar experience once you bring memories up for conscious review. Perhaps you are a teacher in a school that serves underprivileged children in your community. The emotional highs and lows of watching young people with unlimited potential see the light of achievement and then sink back into the comfort of peer pressure instead of breaking free and being themselves is like a roller coaster ride. There may be certain individuals who seem to leave you exhausted once you are no longer in their presence. If you do not take steps to diminish the depletion of your energy and to replenish the stores, you will no longer be in a position to maintain your vitality.

Worst of all is the depletion of mental energy. This is the feeling that "none of my ideas seem to be working." This perception feeds voraciously into a downward spiral. Once mental energy depletes, depression follows, the psychological depth from which it is very difficult to rise.

Our physical reality imposes the laws of entropy and gravity on all matter, including us. Energy is depleted over time in closed systems. This explains why it is never enough to get comfortable or become complacent. If you are not growing, you are disintegrating. You must continually discover, gather, and sequester energy to renew yourself if you wish to live well as long as possible.

Become an Energy Conduit

The renewal of energy occurs when you have a clear purpose and a worthy goal. Personal passion transforms into useable energy and fuels thoughts, feelings, and

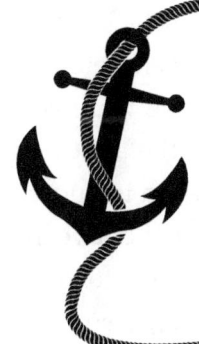

Action Interlude

Recognize people, places and things that deplete your energy. Make a list of 5 for each category: physical, emotional, and mental.

actions. You gather energy from outside sources through the attractive forces of vibrations and resonance. Exercises to strengthen the mental muscles necessary to make this happen appear throughout this book. Now comes the real challenge: How do you sequester this energy so that it is available whenever you need it? What serves as your battery when you want to "go portable"?

Your capacity to store energy and have it available depends upon the smooth interaction of a number of physical, emotional, and mental processes. For example, physical energy is stored in the body as fat. Whether you can retrieve it to serve you depends upon the optimal function of the metabolic processes that break down fat and transport the energy to where the body has a need. Emotional and mental energy are stored within your mind through the interplay of conscious and subconscious, left and right, intellectual and intuitive.

Imagine the Results of More Energy

One of the easiest ways to increase your storage capacity and your ability to access it is to role play or visualize scenarios where a boost of energy would change the outcome. This becomes very apparent in self-defense training. One tactic employed in learning self-defense skills is to visualize yourself protecting someone you love standing behind you so that you are between the attacker and the person you are to protect. For example, an intruder enters a home and the husband positions himself between the intruder and his wife. The husband's passion for his wife gives him a boost of all three forms of energy so that he is more aware of his situation than usual, stronger than usual, and faster than usual. He creates a better chance of saving himself and his wife with proper use of this energy boost.

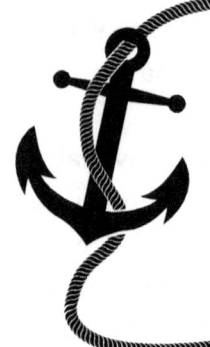

Action Interlude

Think of someone or something you are willing to risk your life to defend. It can be yourself or someone else. Visualize or act out a physical attack on that person's safety where you intervene and "save the day."

Something Larger Than You Are

If you wish to significantly improve the storage and utility of energy, shift your focus from yourself toward a greater cause. Take all of the mental and physical muscles you have been developing and apply them to the success of a cause greater than you. Even if you are approaching your own death, the spirit of helping another will keep you going far longer than dwelling upon your ills. Brendon Burchard is an amazing man who experienced this personally as a college student and captures the lesson in his parable *Life's Golden Ticket: An Inspirational Novel.* If you track the exponential growth in his influence for good in our world, it will inspire you to leave your own footprints.

This final concept closes *Think and Grow Well:* if you want to tap into everlasting energy stores, you must be willing to reach outside of yourself and trust in a plan that is larger than your own existence. The more personal you can make your involvement in the success of this plan, the more active you become mentally, emotionally, and physically. The repetitive activity builds your intellectual faculties, imagination, intuition, memory, will, reason, and perception. The repetitive activity, or practice, increases your emotional capacity and flexibility. The repetitive activity tones all four aspects of your being: body, mind, spirit and awareness, the four strands of your lifeline. The gratitude you express as you feel the joy of your successes, even before they become physical reality, keeps you going. When you take action on all those levels in the service of humanity, you take responsibility for your time on earth, and you shape the future. You think and grow well. Only God knows just how many lives you are saving.

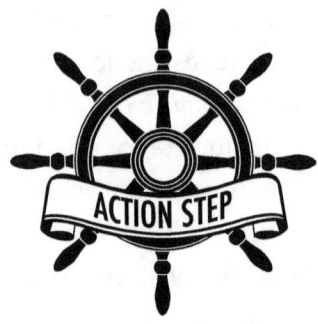

ACTION STEP

Commit to a service project that is in keeping with your life's purpose. It might be feeding the hungry, clothing the poor, mentoring a child that doesn't have strong role models, helping a friend who is hurting, saving a soul. List three things you will do each week to succeed. Follow through with the weekly actions. Journal about how you feel.

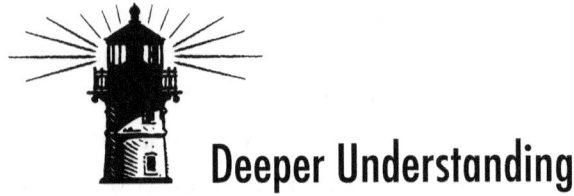

Deeper Understanding

Catch-22, Joseph Heller, Simon and Schuster, New York, NY, 1961.

Positive Energy, Judith Orloff, Harmony Books, New York, NY, 2004.

Read about Joshua and his leadership style in the book of Joshua from the Bible.

Life's Golden Ticket: An Inspirational Novel, Brendon Burchard, Harper Collins, New York, NY, 2008.

The Four-Hour Body, by Timothy Ferriss, Crown Archetype, New York, NY, 2010.

Epilogue

Greg Sterling is mentioned in the dedication. I never met Greg in person. Our family met him through his cooking. His untimely death before the age of 40 was a wake-up call.

Nate is healthy and involved in support services for sports teams and in political activism.

Darcie visited a neurologist and a cardiologist, neither of whom had answers. She tried a new medication. She remains afflicted on occasion, and it is still scary.

Stan is a happy teenager who is known for his honesty, compassion, and courtesy.

Mary is healthy and happy even with continued heath challenges; the most recent was a hip replacement. She sailed through her recovery. She lectures to groups about her experiences and the subsequent deepening of her faith.

Sabrina remains in remission and is in college.

Jerry is dead. When my mother encountered one of his doctors many years later, he commented that Jerry was the one patient who changed his whole outlook on medicine and what was possible.

Sal and her husband enjoy their retirement in the company of their cat and master garden.

My father, Sonny, is a vibrant octogenarian with a wicked sense of humor.

Amy is still scrapbooking and remains trim.

Lee, my mother, is the most energetic woman I have ever known. I asked her once, "It looks like you lost some weight, what is your secret?" She replied, "Work your butt off!" She has fun with that. She planted a row of pumpkins in the summer as she has every year since my son was very young. She also planted a few yellow squash and some loofah squash. Loofah squash are also known as vegetable sponges because of their hard fibrous innards that dry into a natural sponge good for cellulite minimization and for cleaning pots and pans. One day Sonny and I came home from playing a round of golf and were really hungry. She was frying squash. We excitedly enjoyed them. Later on we were walking in the field and I pointed out one of the loofahs growing because she had not grown them before. She started laughing. "I guess that explains why the squash I fried for you was so tough; it was loofah." So much for the crop of natural sponges; we just had them for lunch! I had asked her to consider increasing fiber in her diet. That's one way to have fun with it.

I continue to have interesting encounters with Broca's speech area. The bottom line is, when you learn to surprise Broca, you focus the mind's eye.

After the unique experience of having our first child, my husband and I decided to retire from that labor. Our son continues to be a joy at each age.

Sam's well-being and emotional stability continue to improve. He is currently practicing medicine and is grateful that he did not continue to respond to life's stresses with the negative pattern in which he had trapped himself.

We miss Gene's wry wit and hearty comments, his wood carvings, and his laughter.

Back to Sonny. This book really starts and ends with this

man's stories. He has a great memory and is an engaging storyteller. Concerning aging, he recommends, "Don't get old, kid." Most important, he laughs at himself. He alternates bush hogging the back 40 acres of the farm with playing nine holes of golf on Tuesday through Friday. It works well for him. If you run into him, make sure you aren't taking yourself too seriously. If you are, he will remind you, "Smile every chance you get!"

Now, what's your story?

Send it to me at http://www.thinkandgrowwell.com.

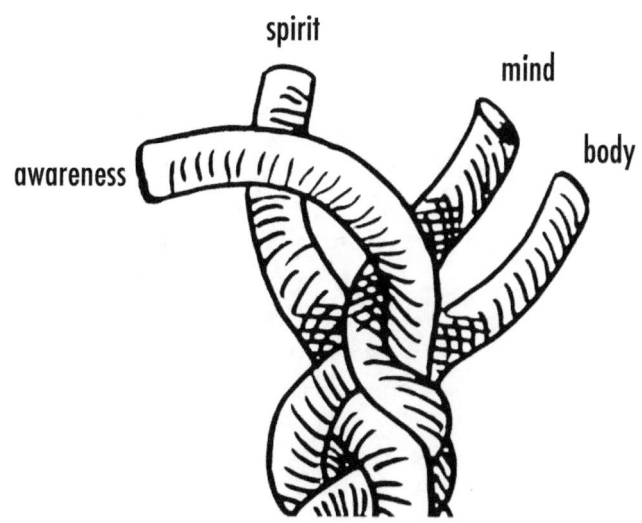

Appendix

Make an Ease-o-Stat™

Physical, digital, and interactive versions are available at http://www.easeostat.com.

Directions:

1. Photocopy the Ease-o-Stat™ pages on card stock.

2. Cut out the circle and the arrow.

3. Affix the arrow to the face of the circle with a brass brad.

4. Align the arrow to the zero mark each morning.

5. Use Ease-o-Stat™ when you feel a strong positive or negative emotion.

6. Grade emotion using a scale of –10 to +10 (or higher for an emotionally charged event). Scales below help gauge your grading.

7. Move cursor to reflect your new score. If score reaches 180 or –180, record score and reset to zero.

8. Record final score at end of day. Add or subtract any recorded scores of 180 or –180 from same day. Your goal is to end each day in the positive value range. After one week, if you are not consistently ending the day with the arrow in the positive, begin adding eustress events so that you end on a positive value.

1_____10
unable to cope   best coping

1_____10
out of control   in control

1_____10
buried   on top

1_____10
scared to death   completely relaxed

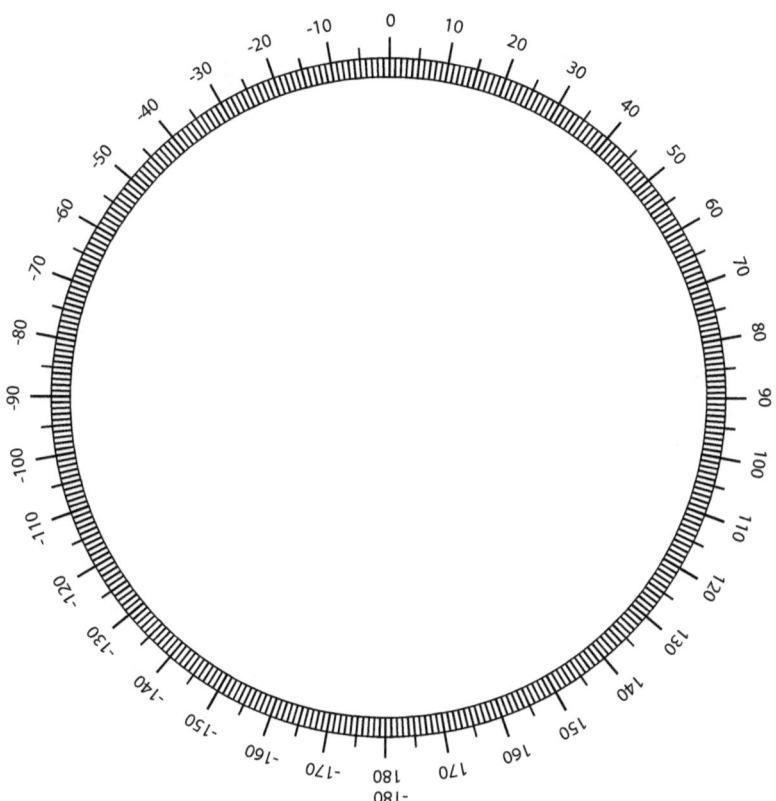

Make an Ease-O-Stat™ 173

Afterword

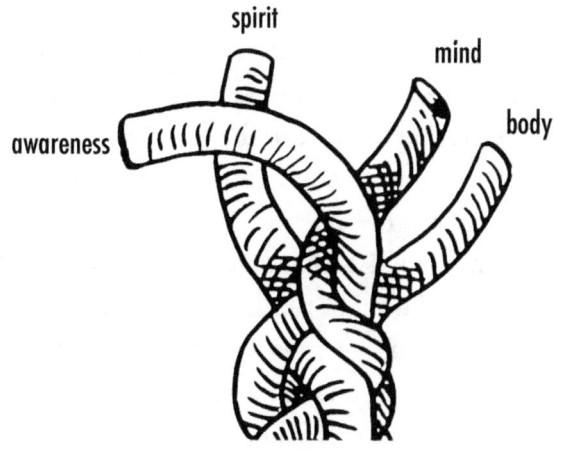

Congratulations! You have just completed *Think and Grow Well,* designed to introduce the idea of trauma preparedness. You braid your lifeline and realize that there are concrete steps that ensure that you enrich your sense of self through any physical crisis. The next question is: will you take these steps regularly so that you are not caught off-guard when dis-ease strikes? A good measure of your willingness to carry out this task is a look back at how actively you participated in the action steps in each chapter. There are many reasons people end up reading *Think and Grow Well* instead of interacting with it. You may more clearly understand how your current paradigms affect your actions. You may be able to identify your mental tattoos.

Here is one way to do it. Carefully go back and review your assessment of each chapter. See which chapters were easy to follow through on and which ones you just wanted to skip. Reflect for a moment on why you think you were either successful or not successful at the activities suggested. List these reasons in your journal. Next, look for patterns in your successes and areas neglected. While you may think that your patterns of action are mere reflections upon my writing, they also reflect your underlying frame of mind as you consider a new idea. Look for what this information says about you. Now that you are aware that a pattern may exist, test it and see if you are using this same lens as you entertain new ideas in other areas of your life. If so, is it serving your life's purpose? If not, take active steps to change it. Often the chapters we find the most repulsive or tedious strike a nerve because they cover an area where personal growth is needed and the work to change seems hard. Our ability to grow in these areas hastens when we identify a goal we are passionate about that requires the change to occur to produce the result we desire.

Thank you for spending a portion of your life studying vitality preparedness, your rope of hope. It is an honor to meet you in this way, and I look forward to meeting you in person or by virtual means. Instead of wishing you good luck, I pray that you are blessed in every endeavor that brings you closer to the achievement of your life's purpose.

Acknowledgements

Grateful acknowledgement to God for the opportunity to share information that will help during challenging periods of life; Dr. Steven Dent, love of my life and sounding board; Dr. Lee Barr, my mentor and inspiration since birth; Ret. Lt. Cmdr. Luther Barr, my father and my favorite storyteller; Richard Dent, one of my greatest teachers and business partner; my second parents, Edith and Gene Dent, the Ginger Rogers and Fred Astaire of dancing with disease gracefully; my friends, relatives, and acquaintances who served as models or inspired the vignettes and action steps; my partners and coworkers at Austin Radiological Association, the best imaging practice in the world; Kendra Sterling who helped me find the space in my life to finish this; my writing coach, Elizabeth Ragland; Brendon Burchard; Dee Burks; Bella Guzmán for layout; Robin Kressbach for illustrations; Bob Proctor, mentor and inspiration; Dr. Susan John for friendship and shared pivotal moments in life; and Carol Provisor, my best friend, who never lets me appear less than my best in public.

Bibliography

Preface

Barr, L., "Mental Tattoos," *DNA of Success Stories*, Zufelt J (ed), Z Publishing, Centennial, CO, 2009.

Introduction

Barr, L., "Mental Tattoos," *DNA of Success Stories*, Zufelt J (ed), Z Publishing, Centennial, CO, 2009.

Novaline R., *Squire's Fundamentals of Radiology*, Harvard University Press, Cambridge, MA, 2004.

Barr, L. (ed.), *Handbook of Pediatric Imaging*, Churchill Livingstone, New York, NY, 1991.

Dubin, D., *Rapid Interpretation of EKGs*, Sixth Edition, Cover Publishing Company, Tampa, FL, 2000.

Chapter 1

Tolstoy, L., *The Death of Ivan Ilyich*, The Editorium, West Valley City, Utah, 2006.

Miller, G., Chen, E., Cole, & S. W., Health psychology: developing biologically plausible models linking the social world and physical health, *Annu Rev Psychol*, 2009; 60:501-24.

Buzan, T. & Buzan, B., *The Mind Map Book*, Penguin Books, New York, NY, 1996.

Frost, R., "Once by the Pacific," *West Running Brook*, Henry Holt, New York, NY, 1928.

Chapter 2

Lewis, C. S., *Mere Christianity*, Harper Collins, New York, NY, 1952.

Fleet, T. C., *Concept Therapy*, Concept Therapy Institute, San Antonio, TX, 1984.

Gladwell, Malcolm., *The Tipping Point*, Bay Back Books, Boston, MA, 2002.

Sheldrake, R. and Lipton, B., "Cells, Minds and Morphic Fields," a dialogue at Seattle, WA, August 2007.

Proctor, B., *You Were Born Rich*, LifeSuccess Productions, Toronto, CA 1997.

Chapter 3

Williams, R., *Thought Particles: Building Blocks of Perceptual Reality; Binary Code of the Mind*, Wizard Academy Press, Buda, TX, 2001.

Baddeley, A., *Essentials of Human Memory*, Psychology Press, East Sussex, Eng 2005.

Marcer, P., Quantum Computation and the Conscious Machine, Why Computers Will Never Be Smarter Than Humans, *AI Soc* 6(1): 88-93, 1992.

Kuhn, T., *The Structure of Scientific Revolutions*, University of Chicago Press, Chicago, IL, 1962.

Covey, S., *The 7 Habits of Highly Effective People*, Simon and Schuster, New York, NY, 1989.

Chapter 4

Sarno, J., *The Mindbody Prescription,* Time Warner Book Group, New York, NY, 1998.

Witek-Janusek, L., Albuquerque, K., Chroniak, K. R., Chroniak, C., Durazo-Arvizu, R., Mathews, H. L., Effect of mindfulness based stress reduction on immune function, quality of life and coping in women newly diagnosed with early stage breast cancer. *Brain Behav Immun.* 2008 Aug;22(6):969-81. Epub 2008 Mar 21.

Janicki-Deverts, D., Cohen, S., Matthews, K.A., Gross, M. D., Jacobs. D. R. Jr., Socioeconomic status, antioxidant micronutrients, and correlates of oxidative damage: the Coronary Artery Risk Development in Young Adults (CARDIA) study. *Psychosom Med.* 2009 Jun;71(5):541-8. Epub 2009 May 4.

Miller, G. E., Cohen, S., Pressman, S., Barkin, A., Rabin, B. S., Treanor, J. J., Psychological stress and antibody response to influenza vaccination: when is the critical period for stress, and how does it get inside the body?, *Psychosom Med.* 2004 Mar-Apr;66(2):215-23.

Chapter 5

Adler, S., *The Art of Acting,* Applause Theatre & Cinema Book Publishers, New York, NY, 2000.

Maltz, M., *Psycho-cybernetics,* Pocket Books, New York, NY, 1969.

Doidge, N. *The Brain That Changes Itself,* Viking Penguin, New York, NY 2007.

Chapter 6

Cercone, D., *MegaLearning*, Nightingale Conant, Chicago, IL.

Gladwell, M. *Outliers*, Little, Brown and Company, New York, NY, 2008.

Holliwell, R., *Working With the Law*, DeVorss & Company, Camarillo, CA, 1938.

Chapter 7

Rosen, S., *My Voice Will Go With You - The Teaching Tales of Milton H. Erickson*, W. W. Norton and Co., New York, NY, 1982.

Zufelt, J. (ed.), *DNA of Success Stories*, Z Publishing, Centennial, CO, 2009.

Lorayne, H., *How to Develop a Super-Power Memory*, Signet Books, New York, NY, 1974.

Hill, N., *Think and Grow Rich*, The Ralston Society, Meriden CT, 1937.

Chapter 8

Carnevale, F. A., Alexander, E., Davis, M., Rennick, J., Troini, R., Daily living with distress and enrichment: the moral experience of families with ventilator-assisted children at home. *Pediatrics*. 2006 Jan;117(1):e48-60.

Raina, P., O'Donnell, M., Rosenbaum, P., Brehaut, J., Walter, S., Russell, D., Swinton, M., Zhu, B., Wood, E., The health and well-being of caregivers of children with cerebral palsy, *Pediatrics*. 2005 Jun;115(6):e626-36.

Gigerenzer, G., *Gut Feelings: the Intelligence of the Unconscious,* Penguin Group, New York, NY, 2007.

Hawkins, D., *Power Vs. Force,* Hay House, Carlsbad, CA, 2002.

Chapter 9

Smith, F. (ed.), *The Daily Bible,* Harvest House Publishers, Eugene, OR, 1999.

Dossey, L., *Healing Words,* Harper Collins, New York, NY, 1993.

Csikszentmihalyi, M., *Flow: The Psychology of Optimal Experience,* Harper and Row, New York, NY, 1990.

Chapter 10

Penick, H., *Harvey Penick's Little Red Book: Lessons and Teachings from a Lifetime of Golf,* Simon and Schuster, New York, NY, 1992.

O'Leary, M. *Perfect Power Golf,* Orlando Florida, 2011

Adams, P. *House Calls, How We Can All Heal the World One Visit at a Time,* Robert D. Reed Publishers, San Francisco, CA 1998.

Chapter 11

Weil, A., *Why Our Health Matters,* Penguin Group, New York, NY, 2009.

Cousins, N., *Anatomy of an Illness as Perceived by the Patient,* W. W. Norton and Company, New York, NY, 1979.

Chapter 12

Dulin, P., and Hill, R., Relationships between altruistic activity and positive and negative affect among low-income older adult service providers. *Aging and Mental Health*, 7, 294-299, 2003.

Bennett, M. and Lengacher, C., Humor and Laughter May Influence Health IV, *Humor and Immune Function, Evidence-Based Complimentary and Alternative Medicine*, 6(2):159-164, 2009.

Paul the Apostle, *I Thessalonians, in The Holy Bible*, American Standard Edition, Nelson Publishing, Nashville, TN, 1901.

Nightingale, E., *Lead the Field,* Nightingale-Conant, Niles, IL, 1960.

Chapter 13

The Holy Bible, American Standard Edition, Nelson Publishing, Nashville, TN, 1901.

Max-Neef, M., *Human Scale Development: Conception, Application and Further Reflections,* The Apex Press, New York. ISBN 0-945257-35-X, 1991.

Robbins, A., *Inner Strength: Harnessing the Power of Your Six Primal Needs,* Free Press, New York, NY, 2010.

Ferriss, T. *The Four-Hour Body*, Crown Archetype, New York, NY, 2010.

Chapter 14

Heller, J., *Catch-22*, Simon and Schuster, New York, NY, 1961.

Schlosser, E., *Fast Food Nation: The Dark Side of the All-American Meal*, Harper Perennial, New York, NY, 2002.

Orloff, J., *Positive Energy*, Harmony Books, New York, NY, 2004.

Joshua, in *The Holy Bible*, American Standard Edition, Nelson Publishing, Nashville, TN, 1901.

Burchard, B., *Life's Golden Ticket: An Inspirational Novel*, Harper Collins, New York, NY, 2008.

Index

affirmation 133
agreement 38, 40, 41, 77
appreciation 70, 139, 140, 141
Broca's speech area 125, 168
collective consciousness 25
Concept Therapy 24, 30, 180
conscious mind 24, 25, 28, 34, 37, 50, 51, 62, 63, 65, 117, 132, 137
death 14, 21, 65, 74, 97, 110, 111, 127, 151, 153, 164, 167
disease xiii, xiv, 2, 8, 9, 11, 20, 25, 26, 29, 48, 49, 50, 53, 54, 56, 61, 62, 65, 69, 72, 76, 78, 84, 88, 111, 125, 127, 129, 131, 175
doubt xii, xiii, 11, 20, 25, 28, 29, 50, 52, 54, 117, 153
ease 49, 51, 53, 56
Ease-o-Stat™ 53, 56, 65, 171
energy 4, 11, 22, 26, 55, 56, 65, 77, 85, 86, 100, 115, 116, 117, 118, 133, 153, 160, 161, 162, 163, 164, 165, 185
environment 26, 35, 62, 77, 78, 117, 131, 133
faith 4, 10, 51, 52, 55, 77, 97, 99, 100, 109, 110, 111, 125, 151, 167
fear 8, 14, 20, 25, 27, 29, 50, 52, 56, 71, 72, 85, 153
genetic programming 25, 26
grace 61, 71, 100, 142, 152, 160
gratitude 70, 100, 109, 110, 138, 139, 140, 141, 142, 165
health xiii, xiv, 4, 11, 35, 49, 50, 65, 77, 78, 84, 90, 96, 97, 100, 125, 127, 128, 129, 130, 131, 132, 133, 139, 161, 179, 182, 183, 184
ignorance 50, 51
imagination 14, 72, 74, 75, 76, 77, 78, 88, 120, 132, 154, 165
intellectual faculties 2, 14, 76, 165
intuition 5, 14, 96, 97, 98, 126, 154, 165
magic 72
mastermind group 73, 90
mastery 12, 65, 71, 74, 90, 108, 120, 121, 151, 159
medical establishment 124

memory 14, 27, 28, 29, 34, 35, 36, 37, 117, 118, 133, 154, 165, 169, 180, 182
mental muscles 14, 154, 163
mental tattoo xiii, 159, 175, 179
morphogenic 26
paradigm 4, 25, 27, 28, 34, 36, 37, 38, 39, 40, 41, 54, 55, 71, 72, 77, 116, 175
paradigms 4
passion xiv, 55, 85, 86, 87, 88, 89, 90, 99, 162, 164, 167
Pasteur 127
patience 96, 97, 99, 100, 154
perception 11, 14, 26, 35, 52, 120, 128, 129, 154, 162, 165
perseverance 10, 96, 97, 99, 100, 115
physical mastery 74, 120
Presence of mind 8, 14
programmed text 5
purpose 5, 47, 50, 51, 53, 54, 55, 78, 142, 162, 176
reason 10, 11, 12, 14, 21, 34, 35, 53, 63, 154, 160, 165, 175, 176
self-image 11, 12, 116
shock xiii, 27, 38, 39, 40, 69, 77, 159
soul 10, 22, 108, 115, 153, 154
spaced repetition 4, 12, 27, 38, 77, 126
spirit xvii, 10, 21, 22, 24, 65, 108, 109, 111, 147, 153, 164, 165
spiritual mastery 108
strategy 28, 37, 131
subconscious 12, 24, 25, 27, 29, 34, 35, 36, 37, 39, 40, 50, 51, 56, 62, 63, 65, 77, 99, 116, 117, 118, 121, 132, 163
terror 65
theory 26
vitality 4, 12, 19, 20, 86, 161, 162, 176
wellness 2, 65, 127, 130, 131, 132, 133
will xiv, 2, 5, 8, 14, 41, 47, 56, 99, 100, 110, 142, 152, 153, 154, 165
worry 19, 20, 25, 26, 28, 29, 50, 52, 86